Environmental Health Criteria 163

CHLOROFORM

First draft prepared by Dr J. de Fouw
National Institute of Public Health and
Environmental Protection, Bilthoven,
Netherlands

Published under the joint sponsorship of
the United Nations Environment Programme,
the International Labour Organisation,
and the World Health Organization

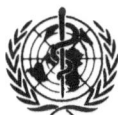

World Health Organization
Geneva, 1994

The **International Programme on Chemical Safety (IPCS)** is a joint venture of the United Nations Environment Programme, the International Labour Organisation, and the World Health Organization. The main objective of the IPCS is to carry out and disseminate evaluations of the effects of chemicals on human health and the quality of the environment. Supporting activities include the development of epidemiological, experimental laboratory, and risk-assessment methods that could produce internationally comparable results, and the development of manpower in the field of toxicology. Other activities carried out by the IPCS include the development of know-how for coping with chemical accidents, coordination of laboratory testing and epidemiological studies, and promotion of research on the mechanisms of the biological action of chemicals.

WHO Library Cataloguing in Publication Data

Chloroform.

  (Environmental health criteria ; 163)

  1.Chloroform - adverse effects   I.Series

  ISBN 92 4 157163 2   (NLM Classification: QV 81)
  ISSN 0250-863X

PRINTED IN FINLAND
94/10218 – VAMMALA – 5500

CONTENTS

ENVIRONMENTAL HEALTH CRITERIA FOR
CHLOROFORM

WHO TASK GROUP ON ENVIRONMENTAL HEALTH CRITERIA FOR CHLOROFORM

Members

Dr M.W. Anders, Department of Pharmacology, University of Rochester, Rochester, New York, USA

Dr D.Anderson, British Industrial Biological Research Association (BIBRA) Toxicology International, Carshalton, Surrey, United Kingdom

Dr R.J. Bull, Washington State University, College of Pharmacy, Pullman, Washington, USA

Dr C.D. Carrington, Food and Drug Administration, Washington DC, USA

Dr M. Crookes, Environment Section, Building Research Establishment, Garston, Watford, United Kingdom

Dr E. Elovaara, Institute of Occupational Health, Department of Industrial Hygiene and Toxicology, Helsinki, Finland

Dr J. de Fouw, Toxicology Advisory Centre, National Institute of Public Health and Environmental Protection (RIVM), Bilthoven, the Netherlands (*Rapporteur*)

Dr M.E. Meek, Environmental Health Directorate, Health Protection Branch, Health and Welfare, Ottawa, Canada (*Chairperson*)

Dr R. Pegram, Environmental Toxicology Division, Health Effects Research Laboratory, US Environmental Protection Agency, Research Triangle Park, North Carolina, USA

Dr S.A. Soliman, Department of Pesticide Chemistry, College of Agriculture and Veterinary Medicine, King Saud University-Al-Qasseem, Bureidah, Saudi Arabia (*Vice-Chairman*)

Dr L. Vittozzi, Istituto Superiore di Sanità, Laboratorio di Tossicologia, Comparata ed Ecotossicologia, Rome, Italy (*Vice-Chairman*)

Dr P.P. Yao, Institute of Occupational Medicine, Chinese Academy of Preventive Medicine, Beijing, China

Representatives of other Organizations

Dr B. Butterworth, International Life Sciences Institute, Risk Science Institute, Washington DC, USA

Secretariat

Dr B.H. Chen, International Programme on Chemical Safety, World Health Organization, Geneva, Switzerland (*Secretary*)

Dr P.G. Jenkins, International Programme on Chemical Safety, World Health Organization, Geneva, Switzerland

Dr C. Partensky, International Agency for Research on Cancer, Lyon, France

NOTE TO READERS OF THE CRITERIA MONOGRAPHS

Every effort has been made to present information in the criteria monographs as accurately as possible without unduly delaying their publication. In the interest of all users of the Environmental Health Criteria monographs, readers are kindly requested to communicate any errors that may have occurred to the Director of the International Programme on Chemical Safety, World Health Organization, Geneva, Switzerland, in order that they may be included in corrigenda.

* * *

A detailed data profile and a legal file can be obtained from the International Register of Potentially Toxic Chemicals, Case postale 356, 1219 Châtelaine, Geneva, Switzerland (Telephone No. 9799111).

* * *

This publication was made possible by grant number 5 U01 ES02617-15 from the National Institute of Environmental Health Sciences, National Institutes of Health, USA, and by financial support from the European Commission.

ENVIRONMENTAL HEALTH CRITERIA FOR CHLOROFORM

A WHO Task Group on Environmental Health Criteria for Chloroform met in Geneva from 15 to 19 November 1993. Dr B.H Chen, IPCS, welcomed the participants on behalf of the Director, IPCS, and the three IPCS cooperating organizations (UNEP/ILO/WHO). The Task Group reviewed and revised the draft document and made an evaluation of risks for human health and the environment from exposure to chloroform.

The first draft was prepared by Dr J. de Fouw of the National Institute of Public Health and Environmental Protection (RIVM), Bilthoven, Netherlands. The second draft was also prepared by Dr J.de Fouw incorporating comments received following the circulation of the first draft to the IPCS Contact Points for Environmental Health Criteria monographs. Dr M.E. Meek (Health and Welfare, Canada) made a considerable contribution to the preparation of the final text.

Dr B.H. Chen and Dr P.G. Jenkins, both members of the IPCS Central Unit, were responsible for the overall scientific content and technical editing, respectively.

The efforts of all who helped in the preparation and finalization of the monograph are gratefully acknowledged.

ABBREVIATIONS

ALAT	alanine aminotransferase
ASAT	aspartate aminotransferase
Brdu	bromodeoxyuridine
DENA	diethylnitrosamine
ENU	ethylnitrosourea
GGTase	γ-glutamyl transpeptidase
LI	labelling index
NOAEL	no-observed-adverse-effect level
NOEC	no-observed-effect concentration
NOEL	no-observed-effect level
NOLC	no-observed-lethal concentration
PBPK	physiologically based pharmacokinetics
SCE	sister-chromatid exchange
SGPT	serum glutamine-pyruvate transaminase
UDS	unscheduled DNA synthesis

1. SUMMARY

Chloroform is a clear, colourless, volatile liquid with a characteristic odour and a burning, sweet taste. It is degraded photochemically, is not flammable and is soluble in most organic solvents. However, its solubility in water is limited. Phosgene and hydrochloric acid may be formed by chemical degradation.

Chloroform is used in pesticide formulations, as a solvent and chemical intermediate. Its use as an anaesthetic and in proprietary medicines is banned in some countries. The commercial production amounted to 440 000 tonnes in 1987. Significant amounts of chloroform are also produced in the chlorination of water and the bleaching of paper pulp.

There are several analytical methods for the analysis of chloroform in air, water and biological materials. The majority of these methods are based on direct column injection, adsorption on activated adsorbent or condensation in a cool trap, then desorption or evaporation by solvent extraction or heating and subsequent gas chromatographic analysis.

It is assumed that most chloroform present in water is ultimately transferred to air, due to its volatility. Chloroform has a residence time in the atmosphere of several months and is removed from the atmosphere through chemical transformation. It is resistant to biodegradation by aerobic microbial populations of soils and aquifers subsisting on endogenous substrates or supplemented with acetate. Biodegradation may occur under anaerobic conditions. The bioconcentration in freshwater fish is low. Depuration is rapid.

Based on estimates of mean exposure from various media, the general population is exposed to chloroform principally in food, drinking-water and indoor air in approximately equivalent amounts. The estimated intake from outdoor air is considerably less. The total estimated mean intake is approximately 2 μg/kg body weight per day. Available data also indicate that water use in homes contributes considerably to levels of chloroform in indoor air and to total exposure. For some individuals living in dwellings supplied with tap water containing relatively high concentrations of chloroform, estimated total intakes are up to 10 μg/kg body weight per day.

Chloroform is well absorbed in animals and humans after oral administration but the absorption kinetics are dependent upon the vehicle of delivery. After inhalation exposure in humans, 60-80% of the inhaled quantity is absorbed. The primary factors affecting the absorption kinetics of chloroform following inhalation are its concentration and species-specific metabolic capacities. It is readily absorbed through the skin of humans and animals and significant dermal absorption of chloroform from water while showering has been demonstrated. Hydration of the skin appears to accelerate absorption of chloroform.

Chloroform distributes throughout the whole body. Highest tissue levels are reached in the fat, blood, liver, kidneys, lungs and nervous system. Distribution is dependent on exposure route; extrahepatic tissues receive a higher dose from inhaled or dermally absorbed chloroform than from ingested chloroform. Placental transfer of chloroform has been demonstrated in several animal species and humans. Chloroform is eliminated primarily as exhaled carbon dioxide. Unmetabolized chloroform is retained longer in fat than in any other tissue.

The oxidative biotransformation of chloroform is catalysed by cytochrome P-450 to produce trichloromethanol. Loss of HCl from trichloromethanol produces phosgene as a reactive intermediate. Phosgene may be detoxified by reaction with water to produce carbon dioxide or with thiols including glutathione or cysteine to produce adducts. The reaction of phosgene with tissue proteins is associated with cell damage and death. Little binding of chloroform metabolites to DNA is observed. Chloroform also undergoes P-450-catalysed reductive biotransformation to produce the dichloromethyl radical, which becomes covalently bound to tissue lipids. A role for reductive biotransformation in the cytotoxicity of chloroform has not been established.

In animals and humans exposed to chloroform, carbon dioxide and unchanged chloroform are eliminated in the expired air. The fraction of the dose eliminated as carbon dioxide varies with the dose and the species. The rate of biotransformation to carbon dioxide is higher in rodent (hamster, mouse, rat) hepatic and renal microsomes than in human hepatic and renal microsomes. Also, chloroform is biotransformed more rapidly in mouse than in rat renal microsomes.

The liver is the target organ for acute toxicity in rats and several strains of mice. Liver damage is characterized mainly by early fatty infiltration and balloon cells, progressing to centrilobular necrosis and then massive necrosis. The kidney is the target organ in male mice of other more sensitive strains. The kidney damage starts with hydropic degeneration and progresses to necrosis of the proximal tubules. Significant renal toxicity has not been observed in female mice of any strain.

Acute toxicity varies depending upon the strain, sex and vehicle. In mice the oral LD_{50} values range from 36 to 1366 mg chloroform/kg body weight, whereas for rats, they range from 450 to 2000 mg chloroform/kg body weight. After a single inhalation exposure of 4 h, liver toxicity was observed in mice and rats at chloroform levels of 490 and 1410 mg/m^3, respectively.

The most universally observed toxic effect of chloroform is damage to the liver. The severity of these effects per unit dose administered depends on the species, vehicle and the method by which the chloroform is administered. The lowest dose at which liver damage has been observed is 15 mg/kg body weight per day administered to beagle dogs in a toothpaste base over a period of 7.5 years. Effects at lower doses were not examined. Somewhat higher doses are required to produce hepatotoxic effects in other species. Although duration of exposure varied in these studies, the no-observed-adverse-effect levels ranged between 15 and 125 mg/kg body weight per day.

Effects in the kidney have been observed in male mice of sensitive strains and in the F-344 rat. Severe effects have been observed in a particularly sensitive strain of male mice at doses as low as 36 mg/kg body weight per day.

Daily 6 h inhalation of chloroform for 7 consecutive days induced atrophy of Bowman's glands and new bone growth in the nasal turbinates of F-344 rats. The no-observed-effect level (NOEL) for these effects was 14.7 mg/m^3 (3 ppm). The significance of these effects is being further investigated in longer-term studies.

Chloroform induced hepatic tumours in mice when adminis-tered by gavage in corn oil at doses in the range of 138 to 477 mg/kg body weight per day. However, when similar doses were administered in drinking-water, there was no effect of chloroform on the yield of hepatic tumours in mice. Moreover, when chloroform was administered in drinking-water as a promoter in initiation/promotion studies, it actually appeared to inhibit the development of diethylnitrosamine-initiated liver tumours in mice. Thus, the vehicle utilized and/or the method in which chloroform is administered is an important variable in its induction of hepatic tumours in mice.

Chloroform induced kidney tumours in rats at doses of 90 to 200 mg/kg body weight per day in corn oil by gavage. However, in this species, results were similar when the chemical was administered in the drinking-water, indicating that the response is not entirely dependent on the vehicle used.

The carcinogenic effects of chloroform on the liver and kidney of rodents appear to be closely related to cytotoxic and cell replicative effects observed in the target organs. The effects on cell replication were found to parallel the modifications of carcinogenic responses to chloroform that were induced by vehicle and mode of administration. The weight of the available evidence indicates that chloroform has little, if any, capability to induce gene mutation or other types of direct damage to DNA. Moreover, chloroform does not appear capable of initiating hepatic tumours in mice or of inducing unscheduled DNA synthesis *in vivo*. On the other hand, hepatic tumours can be efficiently promoted by chloroform when it is administered in an oil vehicle. Consequently, it is likely that, in the case of prolonged administration of chloroform, cytotoxicity followed by cell proliferation is the most important cause for the development of liver and kidney tumours in rodents.

There are some limited data to suggest that chloroform is toxic to the fetus, but only at doses that are maternally toxic.

In general, chloroform elicits the same symptoms of toxicity in humans as in animals. In humans, anaesthesia may result in death due to respiratory and cardiac arrhythmias and failure. Renal tubular necrosis and renal dysfunction have also been observed in humans. The lowest levels at which liver toxicity due to occupational exposure to chloroform has been reported are in the range of 80 to 160 mg/m^3 (with an exposure period of less than 4 months) in one study and in the range of 10 to 1000 mg/m^3 (with exposure periods of 1 to 4 years) in another study. The mean lethal oral dose for an adult is estimated to be about 45 g, but large interindividual differences in susceptibility occur. There is some weight of evidence for an association between exposure to disinfection by-products in drinking-water and colorectal and bladder cancer in some epidemiological studies. However, these studies are compromised by inadequate account of potential confounding factors and other weaknesses. The evidence for the carcinogenicity of chlorinated drinking-water in humans is inadequate. In addition, the disinfection by-products cannot be attributed to chloroform *per se*.

Chloroform is toxic to the embryo-larval stages of some amphibian and fish species. The lowest reported LC_{50} is 0.3 mg/litre for the embryo-larval stages of *Hyla crucifer*. Chloroform is less toxic to fish and *Daphnia magna*. The LC_{50} values for several species of fish are in the range of 18 to 191 mg/litre. There is little difference in sensitivity between freshwater and marine fish. The lowest reported LC_{50} for *Daphnia magna* is 29 mg/litre. Chloroform is of low toxicity to algae and other microorganisms.

The Task Group concluded that the available data are sufficient to develop a tolerable daily intake (TDI) for non-neoplastic effects and risk-specific intakes for carcinogenic effects of chloroform on the basis of studies in animal species; the value will serve as guidance in the development of exposure limits by appropriate authorities. However, it is cautioned that where local circumstances require that a choice must be made between meeting microbiological limits or limits for disinfection by-products such as chloroform, the microbiological quality must always take precedence. Efficient disinfection must *never* be compromised.

Based on the study by Heywood et al. (1979) in which slight hepatotoxicity (increases in hepatic serum enzymes and fatty cysts) was observed in beagle dogs ingesting 15 mg/kg body weight per day in toothpaste for 7.5 years, and incorporating an uncertainty factor of 1000 (x10 for interspecies variation, x10 for intraspecies variation and x10 for use of an effect level rather than a no-effect level and a subchronic study), a TDI of 15 μg/kg body weight per day is obtained.

Based on the available mechanistic data, the approach considered most appropriate for provision of guidance based on mouse liver tumours is division of a no-effect level for cell proliferation by an uncertainty factor. Based on the NOEL for cytolethality and cell proliferation in $B6C3F_1$ mice of 10 mg/kg body weight per day, following administration in corn oil for 3 weeks in the study of Larson et al. (1994a) and incorporating an uncertainty factor of 1000 (x10 for interspecies variation, x10 for intraspecies variation and x10 for severity of effect, i.e. carcinogenicity, and less-than-chronic study), a TDI of 10 μg/kg body weight per day is obtained.

It is recognized that the kidney tumours in rats may similarly be associated with cell lethality and proliferation. However, since data on cell proliferation are not available in the strain where tumours were observed and identified information on cell proliferation and lethality are short-term (one single gavage and 7-day inhalation exposure), it is considered premature to deviate from the default model (i.e. linearized multistage) as a basis for estimation of lifetime cancer risk. The total daily intake considered to be associated with a 10^{-5} excess lifetime risk, based on the induction of renal tumours (adenomas and adenocarcinomas) in male rats in the study by Jorgenson et al. (1985), is 8.2 μg/kg body weight per day.

Levels of chloroform in surface waters are generally low and would not be expected to present a hazard to aquatic organisms. However, higher levels of chloroform in surface water resulting from industrial discharges or spills may be hazardous to the embryo-larval stages of some aquatic species.

2. IDENTITY, PHYSICAL AND CHEMICAL PROPERTIES, AND ANALYTICAL METHODS

2.1 Identity

Chemical formula: $CHCl_3$

Chemical structure:

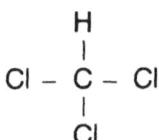

$$Cl - \underset{\underset{Cl}{|}}{\overset{\overset{H}{|}}{C}} - Cl$$

Common name: chloroform

Common synonyms: trichloromethane, methane trichloride, trichloroform, methyl trichloride, methenyl trichloride

CAS chemical name: chloroform

CAS registry number: 67-66-3

RTECS registry number: FS 9100000

2.2 Physical and chemical properties

The most important physical properties of chloroform (IARC, 1979; Windholz, 1983) are given in Table 1.

Chloroform is a clear, colourless, very volatile liquid with a characteristic odour and a burning sweet taste. It is not flammable; however, the substance may be oxidized by strong oxidizing agents with the formation of phosgene and chlorine gas. Pure chloroform is light-sensitive. Reagent grade chloroform therefore usually contains 0.75% ethanol as a stabilizer to avoid photochemical transformation to phosgene and hydrogen chloride (IARC, 1979; Budavari, 1989). In the absence of light this reaction may be catalysed by iron. By the application of stabilizers, such as methanol or ethanol, the auto-oxidation may be prevented since the phosgene is fixed as carbon dioxide dimethyl (or ethyl) ester.

Chloroform stabilized with 0.006% amylenes is now available. This is important for toxicology studies to avoid contamination with by-products that might be formed by reaction with ethanol. The substance is soluble in most organic solvents, such as alcohol, benzene, ether, petroleum ether, carbon tetrachloride, oils and carbon disulfide. Its solubility in water is limited.

Table 1. Physical properties of chloroform

Colour	colourless
Relative molecular mass	119.38
Boiling point at 101.3 kPa	61.3 °C
Melting point	-63.2 °C
Relative density (20 °C)	1.484
Refraction index (Nd 20)	1.4467
Heat capacity (20 °C)	0.979 kJ/kg °C
Critical temperature	263.4 °C
Critical pressure	5.45 MPa
Critical density	500 kg/m^3
Auto-ignition temperature	> 1000 °C
Solubility of chloroform in water (25 °C)	7.5-9.3 g/litre
Heat of combustion	373 kJ/mol
Evaporation heat at standard boiling point	247 kJ/kg
Vapour density (101.3 kPa, 0 °C)	4.36 kg/m^3
Vapour pressure (0 °C)	8 13 kPa
Vapour pressure (20 °C)	21.28 kPa
Stability	air- and light-sensitive, breaks down to phosgene, HCl and chlorine
log K_{ow} (octanol/water partition coefficient)	1.97

Chloroform produces a hydrate, $CHCl_3.17H_2O$, which decomposes at 1.6 °C and 8 kPa. In contact with water, at normal temperatures in the absence of oxygen, chloroform remains stable. It is stable at temperatures up to 290 °C. Heating it in the presence of a diluted caustic solution leads to the formation of formic acid.

The pyrolysis of chloroform vapour at temperatures above 450 °C produces tetrachloroethane, hydrochloric acid and various chlorinated hydrocarbons. In the presence of potassium amalgam or hot copper, acetylene is formed. The reaction with primary amines in an alkaline environment is known as the isonitrile reaction; aromatic hydroxyaldehydes are formed in the presence of phenolates (Reimer-Tiemann reaction). In the Friedel-Crafts reaction, chloroform and benzene produce triphenyl methane. Chlorination of the compound produces tetrachloromethane; bromination of chloroform vapour at 225-275 °C produces CCl_2Br_2 and $CClBr_3$. Chloroform reacts with aluminium bromide to form bromoform ($CHBr_3$). Fluoroform (CHF_3) is produced in the reaction with hydrogen fluoride in the presence of a metallic fluoride as a catalyst. Iodoform (CHI_3) is produced by allowing chloroform to react with ethyl iodide in the presence of aluminium chloride. Unstabilized chloroform reacts with aluminium, zinc and iron. Chloroform mixed with methanolic sodium hydroxide or acetone, in the presence of a base, gives a violent reaction.

2.3 Conversion factors

1 mg chloroform/m³ air = 0.204 ppm at 25 °C and 101.3 kPa (760 mmHg)

1 ppm = 4.9 mg chloroform/m³ air

2.4 Analytical methods

Many analytical methods for the determination of chloroform residues in air, water and biological samples have been reported. Table 2 summarizes some of the procedures used in the literature for sampling and determining chloroform in different media. The detection limits are included in Table 2. Although all of these methods were developed to detect chloroform at very low levels, some of them can be used only in cases where chloroform is present at relatively high levels.

Since chloroform is very volatile, care must be taken while sampling and handling samples to prevent any chloroform from being lost during such procedures. In this case, accuracy depends very much on the repeatability of the method being used. All but one of the methods given in Table 2 use gas chromatographic techniques with electron capture detection (ECD), flame ionisation detection (FID), photo-ionisation detection (PID) or mass spectrometry (MS) for measuring chloroform residues. Only the

Table 2. Sampling and analysis of chloroform

Medium	Sampling method	Analytical method	Detection limit	Sample size	Comments	Reference
Air	aspiration velocity of 28 litres/min, trajectory of 20 m	MIRAN-infrared spectrometer	$300 \ \mu g/m^3$		can be used only when $CHCl_3$ is presented at high levels	Lioy & Lioy (1983)
Air	direct injection	GC with a coulometric ECD	$0.5 \ \mu g/m^3$	5 ml injected	method involves the use of a continuously operating automatic GC monitor	Lasa et al. (1979)
Air	direct injection, calibration gas used for reliability	GC with two ECDs installed serially	$> 0.4 \ \mu g/m^3$ (estimated)	8 ml injected	efficiency followed from signal ratios of the two ECDs	Lillian & Singh (1974)
Air	AIRSCAN/PHOTOVAC direct injection	GC-PID	$0.5 \ \mu g/m^3$	0.05-1 ml	portable machine, suitable for field monitoring	Leveson et al. (1981)
Air	adsorption on activated charcoal, desorption with CS_2	GC-ECD	approximately $0.1 \ \mu g/m^3$	$1 \ m^3/24 \ h$	in 1984 the draft standard NVN 2794 needed to be tested for usefulness	NNI (1984)
Air	adsorption on Porapak-N, desorption with 1-2 ml methanol	GC-ECD	$1 \ \mu g/m^3$	20 litres	advantage of methanol is the absence of a background signal in the ECD	Van Tassel et al. (1981)

Table 2 (contd).

Air	adsorption on Porapak-N, thermal desorption at 200 °C	GC-ECD	estimated to be 0.05 $\mu g/m^3$	0.3-3 litres	confirmation of results by use of GC-MS	Russell & Shadoff (1977)
Air	adsorption on Chromosorb-102, thermal desorption at 150 °C	GC-ECD-FID two detectors positioned in parallel	approximately 0.06 $\mu g/m^3$	1-3 litres		Heil et al. (1979)
Air	adsorption on Tenax, sample rate 10-15 ml/min, thermal desorption and cryofocusing	GC-FID GC-MS	0.08 $\mu g/m^3$	2 ml injected		Kebbekus & Bozzelli (1982)
Air	adsorption on Tenax-GC, cooled with liquid nitrogen, thermal desorption at 270 °C	GC-MS	0.2 $\mu g/m^3$	20 litres		Krost et al. (1982)
Air	adsorption on activated coal, desorption with CS_2, using methylcyclohexane as IS	GC-FID with TCEP, Chromosorb column	0.15 mg detector sensitivity	up to 30 litres can be sampled	these two types of detection appeared to complement each other	Morele et al. (1989)
Air	adsorption on activated coal, desorption with ethanol, using trichloroethylene as IS	GC-ECD with 5% CV17, Chromosorb column	2 μg is minimum quantifiable value			

Table 2 (contd).

Medium	Sampling method	Analytical method	Detection limit	Sample size	Comments	Reference
Air	collection on charcoal, desorption with CS_2 using n-undecane as IS	GC-FID	0.01 mg per sample estimated	up to 15 litres can be sampled	suitable for simultaneous analysis of two or more substances	US NIOSH (1984)
Air	cold trap, heating the cold trap	GC-ECD	0.01 $\mu g/m^3$	30 ml in cold trap	air samples were taken in the stratosphere	Harsch & Cronn (1978)
Air	injection into cold trap, heating the cold trap	GC-MS (SIM)	0.03 $\mu g/m^3$	100 ml in cold trap		Cronn & Harsch (1979)
Air	cold trap after desiccation with magnesium perchlorate, heating the cold trap to 257 °C	GC-PID-ECD-FID, 3 detectors placed sequentially	0.005 $\mu g/m^3$	1 litre	during the process the column is kept at -103 °C (cryofocusing)	Rudolph & Jebsen (1983)
Breath	collection on Tenax GC cartridge, thermal desorption	GC-MS	0.11 $\mu g/m^3$		suitable for quantitative analysis, one sample in 1.5 h	Pellizzari et al. (1985b)
Water	headspace, CH_2Br_2 was used as IS	headspace GC-ECD	0.02 μg/litre	500 μl injected	suitable for routine analysis over a wide range of differently composed river waters	Herzfeld et al. (1989)

Table 2 (contd).

Water	pentane extraction	GC-ECD using 2 mm x 4 mm i.d. column backed with Squalane on Chromosorb P	1 µg/litre	100 ml extracted with 10 ml pentane, 24 litres of extract used for injection	suitable for routine measurements in drinking-water	Oliver (1983)
Water	liquid-liquid extraction with pentane	GC with a Hall electrolyte conductivity detector, Tenax-GC column	0.10 µg/litre	3 µl injected	suitable for routine analyses	Mehran et al. (1984)
Water	direct aqueous injection of sample into GC	GC-ECD with a fused silica capillary column	0.02 µg/litre	2 µl injected	suitable for analyses of halocarbons in the 0.01-10 ppb range	Grob (1984)
Water	direct aqueous injection of sample into GC	GC-ECD with a methyl-silicone fused silica capillary column	0.1 µl/litre	1 µl injected	easy, fast and reliable technique for everyday quality control	Temmerman & Quaghebeur (1990)
Aqueous	diethyl ether extraction with 25 µg p-bromofluoro-benzene as IS	GC-MS with a fused silica capillary column	< 1 µg/litre and recovery efficiency of 0.85	200 ml extracted, extract concentrated to 1 ml, 2 µl injected	suitable for water and homogenized environmental samples	Meier et al. (1985)

Table 2 (contd).

Medium	Sampling method	Analytical method	Detection limit	Sample size	Comments	Reference
Blood	headspace, magnesium sulfate heptahydrate and n-octyl alcohol were added to the plasma	headspace GC-ECD, with Chromosorb W AW column	0.0225 μg/litre (2.5 times standard deviation)	200 μl injected	suitable for direct measurements of $CHCl_3$	Aggazzotti et al. (1987)
Blood	passing inert gas over warmed blood sample, collection on Tenax-GC, thermal desorption	GC-MS	3 μg/litre	1-10 ml	suitable for quantitative analysis of $CHCl_3$ in blood	Pellizzari et al. (1985a)
Blood plasma and stomach contents	diethyl ether extraction (1:1) with 3 different internal standards added to the concentrated extract	GC-MS with a fused silica capillary column	qualitative (no detection limit was given)	1-5 ml, extract concentrated to 1 ml of which 2 μl is injected	suitable for identification of $CHCl_3$ in biological samples	Mink et al. (1983)

Table 2 (contd).

Medium	Sampling method	Analytical method	Detection limit	Sample size	Comments	Reference
Tissue	maceration in water, collection on Tenax-GC, thermal desorption	GC-MS	6 μg/kg	5 g	suitable for semi-quantitative analysis of chloroform in tissues	Pellizzari et al. (1985a)
Urine	pentane extraction	GC-ECD	< 1 μg/litre	2 μl of extract injected	convenient and sensitive means for determining light halogenated hydrocarbons	Youssefi et al. (1978)
Fish	extraction with pentane and isopropanol, bromotrichloromethane used as IS	GC-ECD with a fused silica capillary column	1 μg/kg in fresh material	2 μl injected	extraction efficiency of 67%	Baumann Ofstad et al. (1981)

Abbreviations:

ECD = electron capture detector; FID = flame ionisation detector; GC = gas chromatography; IS = internal standard; MS = mass spectrometry; PID = photo-ionisation detector; SIM = selected ion monitoring first method listed depends on the use of a MIRAN-infrared spectrometer. The sensitivity of this method is very poor.

2.4.1 Sampling and analysis in air

The methods reported in Table 2 for sampling and analysis of chloroform levels in air can be grouped into four different categories.

2.4.1.1 Direct measurement

In this type of procedure, air is aspirated or injected directly into the measuring instrument without pretreatment. Although these methods are simple, they can be used only when chloroform is present in the air at relatively high levels (e.g., urban source areas, see section 5.1.1).

2.4.1.2 Adsorption-liquid desorption

Air samples analysed for their chloroform levels are conducted through an activated adsorbing agent (e.g., charcoal or Porapak-N). The adsorbed chloroform is then desorbed with an appropriate solvent (e.g., carbon disulfide or methanol) and subsequently passed through the gas chromatograph (GC) for measurement.

2.4.1.3 Adsorption-thermal desorption

In this technique, air samples are also passed through an activated absorbing agent (e.g., Tenax-GC, Porapak-Q, Porapak-N or carbon molecular sieve). The adsorbed chloroform is then thermally desorbed and driven into the GC column for determination.

2.4.1.4 Cold trap-heating

In this type of procedure, air samples are injected into a cold trap (liquid nitrogen or liquid oxygen are used for cooling). The trap is then heated while transferring its chloroform content into the packed column of a GC for measurement.

2.4.2 Sampling and analysis in water

Several methods of sampling and analysing water for chloroform content are included in Table 2. In some of these methods, water samples are directly injected into a wide bore or fused silica capillary column to which an ECD is attached. In some other water analysis procedures mentioned in Table 2, the chloroform in the water samples is first extracted by means of a non-polar, non-halogenated solvent (e.g., *n*-pentane). Samples of the obtained extracts are then injected into the GC for determining chloroform. In another procedure, referred to as "close-loop-stripping analysis" (CLSA), chloroform is removed from the water sample by purging it with a large volume of a gas (e.g., nitrogen); the gas is then passed through an adsorption tube and subsequently analysed by GC-MS. Using this latter method, a million-fold concentration can be achieved, so that chloroform can be quantified even at very low levels. A headspace GC technique with ECD has also been used for measuring chloroform levels in water samples (see Table 2).

2.4.3 Sampling and analysis in biological samples

'.4.3.1 Blood and tissues

Several procedures for determining chloroform in blood and tissue samples are presented in Table 2. A headspace GC technique has been used for direct measurement of chloroform in plasma obtained from subjects exposed to low levels in air (Aggazzotti et al., 1987). The second procedure (Kroneld, 1985) depends on liquid-liquid extraction of chloroform from blood samples and subsequent injection of the extract into a GC system for quantification. In the method of Pellizzari et al. (1985a), chloroform is evaporated by passing an inert gas over a warmed plasma or macerated tissue sample with adsorption of the vapour on a Tenax GC column, and is then recovered by thermal desorption and analysed by GC-MS.

'.4.3.2 Urine

Youssefi et al. (1978) measured chloroform concentration in urine using pentane extraction and GC-ECD analysis.

'.4.3.3 Fish

The procedure of Baumann Ofstad et al. (1981) for determining chloroform in fish samples is based on extraction by *n*-pentane and subsequent analysis of the extracts by GC/ECD. It has been reported that the sensitivity of this method is greatly affected by the fat content of the fish samples.

2.4.4 *Sampling and analysis in soil gas*

Kerfoot (1987) determined the level of chloroform in soil gas samples in order to use the results as an indication of ground water contamination by this pollutant. In the procedure used, a 75-ml soil gas sample was drawn from a depth of 1.3 m by means of a sampling probe. The chloroform content of the subsample was directly measured in the field using an on-site GC-ECD. The detection limit for chloroform in soil gas by this method was reported to be 5 parts per billion by volume.

3. SOURCES OF HUMAN AND ENVIRONMENTAL EXPOSURE

3.1 Natural occurrence

Information on the natural occurrence of chloroform has not been identified.

3.2 Anthropogenic sources

3.2.1 Production

3.2.1.1 Direct production levels and processes

Chloroform was prepared, almost simultaneously in 1831, by the action of alkali on chloral (Liebig) and by treating bleaching powder with ethanol or acetone (Soubeirain) (Hardie, 1964). It is currently manufactured in the USA by hydrochlorination of methanol or by chlorination of methane. All chloroform production in Japan and western Europe is by chlorination of methane (IARC, 1979). It can also be manufactured by oxychlorination of methane (ECDIN, 1992).

In the years 1984-1987, the worldwide production of chloroform increased from 360 to 440 kilotonnes (see Table 3).

3.2.1.2 Indirect production

An important contribution to the total emission of chloroform is made through its formation from other substances. In particular the reaction of chlorine with organic compounds may produce substantial quantities of chloroform. With respect to the formation of chloroform in the aquatic medium, it may be assumed that the quantities produced are ultimately emitted totally to the atmosphere.

The following sources are known to contribute to the formation and emission of chloroform:

- Paper bleaching with chlorine (US EPA, 1984; Rosenberg et al., 1991).

- Chlorination of drinking-water (US EPA, 1984).

Table 3. Chloroform production and production capacity expressed in kilotonnes over a period of 15 years (1973-1988)

Country	Year	Production	Capacity
USA	1975	118	-
	1980	160	-
	1984	179	-
	1985	-	200
	1986	191	-
	1987	204	-
	1988	-	218
Japan	1984	46	-
	1985	-	55
	1987	55	-
	1988	-	60
Italy	1973	13	-
	1988	-	55
France	1973	14	-
	1987	45	-
	1988	-	55
Federal Republic of Germany	1973	22	-
Netherlands	1973	8	-
Belgium	1973	15	-
European Economic Community	1979	80	-
	1980	95	-
	1982	-	155
	1984	130	-
	1985	-	160
	1987	150	-
	1988	-	200
World	1984	360	-
	1987	440	-
	1988	-	500

From: ECDIN (1992)

- Chlorination of swimming pool water (Bätjer et al., 1980). A study on emissions in indoor public swimming pools in Bremen (Germany) revealed that an average of 10 g chloroform may be produced daily.

- Chlorination of cooling water. The quantity of chloroform formed depends on a vast range of factors, such as acidity and the concentration of organic materials.

- Chlorination of waste water.

- Exhaust emissions from traffic. The exhaust fumes of vehicles have been demonstrated to contain chloroform; this originates from the decomposition of 1,2-dichloroethane, which is added to petrol as a lead scavenger (US EPA, 1984). Rem et al. (1982) estimated the amount of chloroform to be 1% of the amount of 1,2-dichloroethane added.

- Decomposition of trichloroethene in the atmosphere. At high concentrations (1 ppm) in the presence of light and NO_2, 1% was estimated to be converted (Appleby et al., 1976). US EPA (1984) estimates this emission to be 780 tonnes/year in the USA.

- Decomposition of 1,1,1-trichloroethane has also been suggested as a source (van der Heijden et al., 1986).

Appleby et al. (1976) found that, at relatively high concentrations (1 ppm), trichloroethene may yield about 1% chloroform under the influence of light and NO_x. The estimated production of chloroform from trichloroethene is, at most, about 3 x 10^6 kg/year; in reality the value is likely to be lower.

A possible source of chloroform (van der Heijden et al., 1986) is its production from 1,1,1-trichloroethane via the photolysis of the formed chloral. The increase of chloroform levels in the southern hemisphere since 1974 (from 3 to 11 ppt), is in accordance with the increase in the levels of 1,1,1-trichloroethane during the same period (from 25 to 116 ppt).

2.1.3 Emissions from direct production and use

Almost all of the emissions arise from production, storage, transit and use.

Estimations of emission factors for the production of chloroform range from 0.51 kg chloroform/tonne chloroform (controlled) to 3.35 kg chloroform/tonne chloroform (uncontrolled) (US EPA, 1984). The Federal Office of the

Environment (1981) published a higher emission factor of 18 kg chloroform/tonne chloroform.

With respect to emissions of chloroform in the production of chlorodifluoromethane, emission factors ranging from 0.077-0.33 kg chloroform/tonne chlorodifluoromethane (controlled) to 0.59-2.5 kg chloroform/tonne chlorodifluoromethane (uncontrolled) have been reported (US EPA, 1984). The Federal Office of the Environment (1981) reported an emission factor of 8 kg chloroform/tonne chlorodifluoromethane.

3.2.1.4 Emissions from indirect production

Significant losses of chloroform can also be expected from indirect production of chloroform during the chlorination of water and paper pulp. Data on the magnitude of such emissions have not been identified.

3.2.2 Uses

In the period 1980-1987, the use of chloroform increased in the USA from 170 to 200 kilotonnes and in the EEC from 90 to 110 kilotonnes. The use in Japan was 70 kilotonnes in 1987 (ECDIN, 1992). Chloroform is used in pesticide formulations, in the production of other chemicals, and as a solvent. More than 80% of the produced chloroform is used for the production of chlorodifluoromethane (ECDIN, 1992). This use is likely to decrease in the future due to planned phase-out under the Copenhagen Amendment to the Montreal Protocol (1992). Chloroform was formally used as an anaesthetic (IARC, 1979).

In many countries the use of chloroform is banned as an ingredient (active or inactive) in human drug and cosmetic products (US FDA, 1976). However any drug product containing chloroform in residual amounts, resulting from its use as a processing solvent in manufacture or as a by-product from the synthesis of an ingredient, is not considered to contain chloroform as an ingredient (US FDA, 1976). Chloroform is registered for use in the USA as an insecticidal fumigant for stored barley, corn, oats, popcorn, rice, rye, sorghum and wheat (US EPA, 1971).

4. ENVIRONMENTAL TRANSPORT, DISTRIBUTION AND TRANSFORMATION

4.1 Transport and distribution between media

4.1.1 Transport

Owing to its relatively high volatility, chloroform is preferentially transferred from surface water to air. The experimental half-life of chloroform in water (1 ppm solution with a depth of 6.5 cm at 25 °C) was found to be 18.5 to 25.7 min in a volatilization study by Dilling (1977). In the case of ground waters, however, exchange with the atmosphere may not take place as readily (Uchrin & Mangels, 1986).

4.1.2 Distribution

Adsorption - desorption

Uchrin & Mangels (1986) described the sorptive behaviour of chloroform to solids from the Cohansey (90% sand, 8% silt, 2% clay, 4.4% organic matter) and Potomac-Raritan-Magothy (70.4% sand, 24% silt, 5.6% clay, 2.2% organic matter) aquifer systems, located in the southern New Jersey coastal plain. The fact that chloroform showed a greater tendency to adsorb to the Cohansey material than to the Potomac-RM material might be explained by the difference in organic matter content. The organic carbon normalized partition coefficient K_{oc} was calculated by Uchrin & Mangels (1986) in two ways and appeared to be 57.5 or 70.8. These values are in agreement with the K_{oc} values of 86.7 and 63.4 obtained for Cohansey and Potomac-RM aquifer solids, respectively. Results from the consecutive desorption experiments suggest that the sorption processes in the systems used are not completely reversible.

4.1.3 Removal from the atmosphere

Since no data on the removal rate of chloroform through deposition are available, the values are based on estimates and calculations. These values, however, differ widely. The estimated half-lives range from 92 to 900 years for wet deposition and from 20 days to 22 years for dry deposition.

The calculated half-lives for chloroform degradation are reported to be approximately 100 to 180 days. Reaction with hydroxyl radicals is likely to be the only mechanism for the decomposition of chloroform in the atmosphere (van der Heijden et al., 1986). Cox et al. (1976) determined the relative rate constant for chloroform in comparison with methane in smog chamber studies to be $K = 270$ ppm^{-1} min^{-1}. However, it is known that the decomposition of chlorinated hydrocarbons may lead to intermediary products that can accelerate the decomposition process. Dimitriades et al. (1983) noted that, in a smog chamber, tetrachloroethene is degraded more rapidly than might be expected on the basis of the reaction rate constant. Another drawback of the method of Cox et al. (1976) is the false assumption that the decomposition of hydrocarbons always leads to a transformation of two NO molecules for each carbohydrate molecule transformed. The absolute rate constants determined by Howard Carleton & Evenson (1976) and by Davis et al. (1976) are in agreement with each other, and are $K_{(OH)} = 170 \pm 20$ ppm^{-1} min^{-1} and $K_{(OH)} = 160 \pm 10$ ppm^{-1} min^{-1}, respectively. Based on these rate constants of 170 and 160 ppm^{-1} min^{-1}, a half-life of approximately 60 days can be calculated for the decomposition of chloroform in the atmosphere, assuming a 12-h daytime average hydroxyl radical concentration of 2×10^{-15} mol/litre (Lyman et al., 1982).

When chloroform is irradiated in the presence of chlorine, a rapid reaction takes place, resulting in the formation of radicals. At later stages the trichloromethyl radical may also be formed from the reaction of $CHCl_3$ with the hydroxyl radical. The trichloromethyl radical subsequently reacts with oxygen to form the trichloromethyl peroxyl radical, which ultimately leads to the formation of phosgene (Spence et al., 1976). This is a possible mechanism for the formation of phosgene in ambient air from chlorination.

4.2 Biotic degradation

Strand & Shippert (1986) reported that chloroform is resistant to biodegradation by aerobic microbial communities of soils and aquifers subsisting on endogenous substrates or supplemented with acetate (Wilson et al., 1981; Bouwer & McCarty 1983). Strand & Shippert (1986) used Indianola sandy loam to study the oxidation of chloroform to carbon dioxide in natural gas-enriched soils. It appeared that some chloroform was oxidized by soils that were exposed to cylinder air only, but that the rate in natural gas-enriched soils was four times higher. Chloroform oxidation rates increased with increasing chloroform concentrations up to 5 $\mu g/g$ soil (see Table 4). Chloroform oxidation continued up to 31 days but was inhibited by acetylene and higher concentrations of methane, indicating that methane-oxidizing bacteria may catalyse chloroform oxidation.

Table 4. Effect of chloroform concentration on chloroform oxidation

Applied chloroform concentration ($\mu g/g$ soil)	Chloroform oxidized (ng/5 g soil)[a]
0.02	2.8 ± 1.3
0.11	8.9 ± 7.7
0.55	3.2 ± 7.7
1.09	11.1 ± 3.6
5.47	20.7 ± 9.6

[a] Measured during an 8-day incubation in 5 g of aerobic soil acclimated to natural gas

Bouwer et al. (1981) found significant degradation of chloroform in seeded cultures, relative to controls, at initial concentrations of 16 and 34 $\mu g/litre$. At a high initial chloroform concentration of 157 $\mu g/litre$, degradation was less evident, although there was a gradual reduction in chloroform concentration relative to the sterile controls. The anaerobic degradation appeared to be the result of biological action, although a combination of chemical and biological mechanisms is also possible.

Chloroform can be degraded by reductive dehalogenation under anaerobic conditions. It can be reduced by pure cultures of the methanogen *Methanobacterium thermoautotrophicum* or the sulfate-reducing bacterium *Desulfobacterium autotrophicum* (Egli et al., 1987). In anaerobic sediments, chloroform is probably degraded to carbon dioxide via a carbene mechanism (Bouwer & McCarty, 1983).

Van Beelen & Van Keulen (1990) studied the degradation of radiolabelled chloroform under natural conditions in microcosm experiments. In these experiments, the degradation was monitored by the appearance of radiolabelled carbon dioxide rather than by the disappearance of chloroform. This has the advantage that sorption, which can also lead to disappearance of chloroform, does not interfere with the measurements. At a concentration of 4 µg chloroform/litre, the degradation followed first-order kinetics, with half-lives of 12 days at 10 °C and 2.6 days at 20 °C. At a concentration of 400 µg chloroform/litre, the degradation rate increased with time. After 63 days, the final percentages of label in carbon dioxide and chloroform happened to be similar to the values of the 4-µg/litre experiment. At the other time intervals the percentages of formed carbon dioxide were lower at the higher chloroform concentration. Evidently the degradation rate of chloroform at 400 µg/litre increases with time due to adaptation of the bacteria in the sediment.

4.3 Bioaccumulation

Anderson & Lusty (1980) determined bioaccumulation in four species of fish (*Salmo gairdneri*, *Lepomis macrochirus*, *Micropterus salmoides* and *Ictalurus punctatus*). The bioaccumulation factor (on a fresh weight basis) appeared to be maximal in *Salmo gairdneri* (approximately 10). Depuration was complete in this species within 48 h. A similar value of 6 (whole body; fresh weight) in *Lepomis macrochirus* was reported by Veith et al. (1978).

5. ENVIRONMENTAL LEVELS AND HUMAN EXPOSURE

5.1 Environmental levels

5.1.1 Ambient air

An overview of the concentrations of chloroform measured in areas far from anthropogenic sources is presented in Table 5.

Table 5. Reported concentrations of chloroform in remote areas
(From: van der Heijden et al., 1986).

Northern hemisphere			Southern hemisphere		
Locality	Year	Level (μg/m³)	Locality	Year	Level (μg/m³)
Cork, Ireland	1974	0.133	Cape Town	1974	< 0.015
Pacific Ocean (N.W.)	1976	0.044	South Africa	1977	< 0.015
California	1976	0.085	Pacific Ocean 30-40°S, 138-146°E	1981	0.105
California	1977	0.100	South Pole	1981	0.08
Kansas	1978	0.08	Australia	1981	0.110
Marshall Islands	1981	0 130	Samoa	1981	0.110
Cape Meares, Oregon	1981	0 225	Eastern Pacific 0-40°S	1981	0.055
Pt Barrow, Alaska	1981	0.195			
Hawaii	1981	0.160			
Eastern Pacific 0-40°N	1981	0.105			

Chloroform levels in urban centres may be elevated in comparison with concentrations in remote areas. As in the case of other countries, levels in ambient air in remote areas of the USA range from 0.1 to 0.25 μg/m³. In urban and source-dominated areas, concentrations are 0.3-9.9 μg/m³ and 4.1-110 μg/m³, respectively (ATSDR, 1991). The population-weighted mean concentration of chloroform at 17 urban sites sampled across Canada in 1989 was 0.2 μg/m³ (Environment Canada, 1991).

Su & Goldberg (1976) reported chloroform levels of 1-15 $\mu g/m^3$ in Japanese and European cities. Hourly average concentrations of chloroform in the Netherlands, determined during 1979-1981, were generally 0.15 $\mu g/m^3$ or less (estimated detection limit), the maximum value being 10 $\mu g/m^3$ (Den Hartog, 1980, 1981). Average concentrations of chloroform during 1990 in four German cities (Berlin, Tübingen, Freudenstadt and Leipzig) ranged from 0.26 to 0.9 $\mu g/m^3$; the maximum value was 30 $\mu g/m^3$ detected in Tübingen (Toxicology and Environmental Health Institute of Munich Technical University, 1992).

5.1.2 Indoor air

In a study conducted by the US EPA, volatile organic compounds including chloroform were determined in breath, breathing zone air, fixed outdoor air, drinking-water and some foodstuffs of populations in the USA (Wallace, 1987). The observed increase in the median concentration of indoor versus outdoor air (approximately 85%) was considered to be consistent with assumptions concerning daily water use and likely release of chloroform from water into air (Wallace, 1987). Based on a survey conducted in 1981 in the Federal Republic of Germany, Bauer (1981) reported that levels of chloroform may be higher in kitchens where foodstuffs and water are heated.

Taketomo & Grimsrud (1977) reported average indoor air concentrations of chloroform to be 0.3 $\mu g/m^3$ in a family house and 1.0-3.4 $\mu g/m^3$ in an apartment in Montana, USA, compared to 0.2 $\mu g/m^3$ in outdoor air. In a nationwide survey of 757 randomly selected one-family houses in Canada sampled over a 10-month period in 1991, the mean level of chloroform in indoor air was 4.1 $\mu g/m^3$; the maximum value was 69 $\mu g/m^3$ (Otson et al., 1992). Ullrich (1982) reported comparable concentrations in indoor air (1-3 $\mu g/m^3$) in Germany, although data on outdoor air levels in the vicinity were not presented. Taketomo & Grimsrud (1977) reported indoor air chloroform concentrations of between 2 and 10 $\mu g/m^3$ in buildings other than residences, e.g., restaurants and shops.

Higher levels of chloroform occur in the air of enclosed swimming pools, resulting from water chlorination with sodium hypochlorite and subsequent release to air. Over a period of eleven months, the levels of chloroform directly above the water surface in indoor public swimming pools in Bremen, Germany, ranged from 10 to 380 $\mu g/m^3$, with an average of about 100 $\mu g/m^3$

(Bätjer et al., 1980; Lahl et al., 1981a). Ullrich (1982) reported a similar mean value in four public swimming pools in Germany. Chloroform levels in the air of enclosed swimming pools are a function of several factors such as the degree of ventilation, the level of chlorination, water temperature, the degree of mixing at the water surface, and the quantity of organic precursors present (Lahl et al., 1981a).

5.1.3 Water

5.1.3.1 Sea water

The maximum concentration of chloroform determined in a survey of bay water at 172 locations was 1 μg/litre (Pearson & McConnell, 1975). Reported levels in the open ocean (east Pacific) and off the coast of California were 0.015 μg/litre and 0.009-0.012 μg/litre, respectively (Su & Goldberg, 1976).

5.1.3.2 Rivers and lakes

Concentrations of chloroform in surface water vary, depending upon the proximity to industrial sources. Concentrations of up to 394 μg/litre have been reported in rivers in highly industrial cities (Ewing et al., 1977; Pellizzari et al., 1979). Levels in areas not affected heavily by industrial sources ranged from trace to 22 μg/litre (Ohio River Valley Water Sanitation Commission, 1980, 1982). Concentrations in river water in Germany and Switzerland ranged from about 0.01 to 30 μg/litre (Reynolds & Harrison, 1982). Average concentrations of chloroform detected in 1989 in German rivers ranged from 0.131 to 3.17 μg/litre, with a maximum level of 5.1 μg/litre detected in the River Main (Toxicology and Environmental Health Institute of Munich Technical University, 1992).

5.1.3.3 Rain water

Kawamura & Kaplan (1983) measured 0.25 μg chloroform/litre in Los Angeles rain water samples taken in the spring of 1982.

5.1.3.4 Waste water

Based on two to four samplings at each of 37 plants (22 branches of industry), Van Luin & Van Starkenburg (1984) detected chloroform mainly in the waste water of flavouring and pharmaceutical industries at concentrations of 300 and 16 μg/litre, respectively. Concentrations were lower in the waste water of slaughter-houses, laundries, and textile, rubber and dye industries. In waste-water discharges from the treatment of sewage and industrial wastes in the USA, chloroform was detected at concentrations ranging from 7.1 to 12.1 μg/litre (Europ-Cost, 1976).

5.1.3.5 Ground water

Concentrations of chloroform in ground water vary widely, depending principally on proximity to hazardous waste sites (ATSDR, 1993). Chloroform was detected at levels ranging from 11 to 866 μg/litre in samples from 5 out of 6 monitoring wells drilled 64 m apart in a direction perpendicular to the northward flow of ground water at a contaminated site in Pittman, Nevada, USA (the depth of unconfined ground water was 2 to 4 m at this selected site) (Kerfoot, 1987). In a survey of potentially contaminated sites conducted by the US EPA, chloroform was detected at 45% of the sites. The median and maximum concentrations were 1.5 and 300 μg/litre, respectively (Westrick et al., 1989). In 8 out of 29 deep wells in the Netherlands sampled at least twice since 1980 at several depths (± 10 and 25 m below ground level), chloroform was detected (limit of detection, 0.1 μg/litre) (Van der Heijden et al., 1986).

5.1.3.6 Drinking-water

Chloroform can be formed from naturally occurring organic compounds during the chlorination of drinking-water with the rate and degree of formation being a function primarily of the concentrations of chlorine and humic acid, temperature and pH. Levels vary seasonally, the concentrations generally being greater in summer than winter.

Stander (1980) detected chloroform in 16 out of 20 tap water samples from the USA and western Europe. The highest concentration was 60 μg/litre.

In a national survey of 450 community water supplies in the USA sampled in 1978, chloroform was detected in 94% of surface water supplies and 34% of ground-water supplies. Median concentrations in surface and ground-water supplies were 60 μg/litre and less than the detection limit (0.5 μg/litre), respectively (Brass et al., 1981). Finished drinking-water collected in 1988 from 35 sources in the USA, of which 10 were located in

California, sampled in all four seasons (spring, summer and autumn in 1988 and winter in 1989), contained median concentrations of chloroform ranging from 9.6 to 15 μg/litre. The overall median for all four seasons was 14 μg/litre (Krasner et al., 1989). In a survey conducted in the USA between October 1987 and March 1989, the mean concentration in finished water for surface water systems serving more than 10 000 people was 38.9 μg/litre (90th percentile, 74.4 μg/litre). The comparable mean value in the distribution system was 58.7 μg/litre (US EPA, 1992).

In a national survey of the water supplies of 70 communities in Canada conducted during the winter of 1976/1977, concentrations of chloroform in treated water of the distribution system 0.8 km from the treatment plant averaged 22.7 μg/litre (Williams et al., 1980). Concentrations at 10 different locations in southern Ontario sampled in the early 1980s were 4.5 to 60 μg/litre in water leaving the treatment plant and 7.1 to 63 μg/litre one mile from the plant (Oliver, 1983).

Chloroform levels in drinking-water in 100 German cities sampled in 1977 ranged from < 0.1 to 14.2 μg/litre and averaged 1.3 μg/litre. Concentrations vere similar in other surveys conducted in Germany in the late 1970s and early 1980s (Lahl et al., 1981a). Concentrations of chloroform in chlorinated samples of Rhine river water were 9 μg/litre, compared to 0.1 μg/litre in untreated water from the river (Zoeteman et al., 1982)

In Japan, chloroform was detected at concentrations of 18 and 36 μg/litre in drinking-water (Kajino, 1977).

5.1.4 Soil

No data on concentrations of chloroform in uncontaminated soil have been identified. Chloroform has been detected, however, in 9.9% of hazardous waste sites in the USA; the median concentration was 12.5 μg/kg (ATSDR, 1993).

5.1.5 Foodstuffs

Chloroform has been detected in several foodstuffs, in particular in decaffeinated coffee (20 μg/kg), olive oil (28 μg/kg), pork (10 μg/kg) and sausages (17 μg/kg). Occasionally, concentrations were higher: up to 80 μg/kg in coffee and 90 μg/kg in sausages. Levels of 1 to 10 μg/kg have been detected in flour products, potatoes, cod liver oil, margarine, lard, fish, mussels and milk; levels in most foodstuffs, however, were less than 1 µg/kg (Bauer, 1981).

Daft (1988) reported that chloroform was detected in about 90 of 300 samples in a market-basket survey of 231 "table ready" foodstuffs (prepared and cooked as normally served) in the USA, most often in fat-containing samples. In a later account, it was reported that 2 to 830 µg chloroform/kg food was detected in 68% of 549 samples of foodstuffs obtained in a market-basket survey, grouped as fat, non-fat, grain-based and non-grain-based (average of 71 µg/kg) (Daft, 1989).

Entz et al. (1982) did not detect chloroform in composite samples of meat/fish/poultry or in composite samples of oil/fat in 39 different foods in the USA, although it should be noted that the quantification limits were higher (18 to 28 µg/kg) than those in the studies described above. However, the authors did detect chloroform at a concentration of 17 µg/litre in the composite of dairy foods.

Concentrations of chloroform in soft drinks range from 3 to 50 µg/litre, with levels for cola being at the upper end of the range (Abdel-Rahman, 1982; Entz et al., 1982; Wallace et al., 1984).

5.2 General population exposure

Based on estimates of mean exposure from various media, the general population is exposed to chloroform principally in food (approximately 1 µg/kg body weight per day), drinking-water (approximately 0.5 µg/kg body weight per day) and indoor air (0.3 to 1 µg/kg body weight per day) in approximately equivalent amounts. Estimated intake from outdoor air is considerably less (0.01 µg/kg body weight per day). For some individuals living in dwellings supplied with tap water containing relatively high concentrations of chloroform, exposures may be as high as 10 µg/kg body weight per day.

5.2.1 Outdoor air

Based on a daily inhalation volume for adults of 22 m³, a mean body weight for males and females of 64 kg, the assumption that 4 out of 24 h are spent outdoors (WHO, in press), and the mean levels of chloroform in ambient air in cities presented in section 5.1.1 (0.2 µg/m³), mean intake of chloroform from ambient air for the general population is estimated to be 0.01 μg/kg body weight per day.

5.2.2 Indoor air

Based on a daily inhalation volume for adults of 22 m³, a mean body weight for males and females of 64 kg, the assumption that 20 out of 24 h are spent indoors (WHO, in press), and the mean levels of chloroform in indoor air presented in section 5.1.2 (1 to 4 μg/m³), mean intake of chloroform from indoor air for the general population is estimated to be 0.3 to 1.2 μg/kg body weight per day.

Aggazzotti et al. (1990) determined levels of chloroform in samples of plasma of swimmers and visitors taken "a few minutes after" exposure at indoor swimming pools with water chloroform concentrations of 16.9–47 μg/litre. Concentrations of chloroform in the plasma of all 127 subjects who attended the pools averaged 0.82 μg/litre and ranged from 0.1 to 3 μg/litre, whereas in the plasma samples of 40 nonexposed subjects, chloroform was not detected (limit of quantification, 0.1 μg/litre). The mean level of chloroform in the plasma was significantly higher in swimmers who breathed under stress for a long time directly at the surface of the water (training for competitions).

Individuals may be exposed to elevated concentrations of chloroform (from chlorinated tap water) during showering (Jo et al., 1990a,b).

After showering for 10 min in water containing 5 to 36 μg chloroform/litre, the concentrations of chloroform in the breath of six individuals ranged from 6.0 to 21 μg/m³, while none was detected (detection limit 0.86 μg/m³) in any of the samples of breath collected prior to a shower (Jo et al., 1990b). Based on assumptions of an absorption efficiency from the respiratory tract of 0.77, a breathing rate of 0.014 m³/min for a 70-kg adult, a shower air concentration of 157 μg chloroform/m³ and a ratio of body burden resulting from dermal exposure to that of inhalation exposure of 0.93, the authors estimated that the average intake of chloroform (inhalation and dermal absorption) was 0.5 μg/kg body weight per shower for a person weighing 70 kg.

Based on a review of relevant estimates, Maxwell et al. (1991) concluded that the ratio of the dose of chloroform received over a lifetime from inhalation to that received from ingestion of drinking-water is probably in the range of 0.6-1.5 but could be as high as 5.7. The ratio of the dose received dermally compared to that received orally over a lifetime from drinking-water was considered to be approximately 0.3 but could be as high as 1.8.

5.2.3 Drinking-water

Based on a daily volume of ingestion for adults of 1.4 litres and a mean body weight for males and females of 64 kg (WHO, in press), and the mean levels of chloroform presented in section 5.1.3 (generally < 20 µg/litre), estimated mean intake of chloroform from drinking-water for the general population is less than 0.5 µg/kg body weight per day. As discussed by Bauer (1981), actual levels of exposure may be less than those estimated on the basis of mean levels in drinking-water since most of the chloroform would be expelled from drinking-water that is heated before consumption (tea, coffee, soups, sauces). For example, approximately 96% of the total volatile halogenated hydrocarbon fraction was eliminated in water boiling for 5 min, whereas 50-90% was eliminated upon heating at 70-90 °C (Bauer, 1981). It should be noted, however, that owing to the wide variations in concentrations of chloroform in water supplies, intake from drinking-water could be considerably greater than estimated here for some segments of the general population.

5.2.4 Foodstuffs

Based on a daily volume of ingestion of solid foodstuffs for reference adults of 1.536 kg and a mean body weight for males and females of 64 kg (WHO, in press), and the mean level and percentage detection of chloroform in foodstuffs in a market-basket survey reported by Daft (1989) (section 5.1.5), estimated daily intake of chloroform from foodstuffs is approximately 1 µg/kg body weight per day.

5.3 Occupational exposure during manufacture, formulation or use

Workers may be exposed to chloroform during, for example, the production of chloroform itself, the synthesis of substances derived from chloroform (for example chlorodifluoromethane), the use of chloroform as a solvent in bleaching of paper, and in sewage treatment facilities. Based on a national survey conducted from 1981 to 1983, NIOSH estimated that approximately

96 000 workers in the USA are potentially exposed to chloroform (ATSDR, 1993).

Chloroform is used as a solvent both industrially and in the laboratory; several studies on concentrations in laboratories have been published. Taketomo & Grimsrud (1977) reported levels of 2.3-8.6 mg/m^3 in three laboratories in Montana, USA. In an office situated in the same building but distant from the laboratories, levels were similar; this was attributed to transfer through the air-conditioning system. Levels found by NIOSH in laboratories ranged from 0.5 to 24.9 mg/m^3 (Salisbury, 1982). Time-weighted (4 h) average levels during laboratory practicals were 0-375 mg/m^3 (Hertlein, 1980).

Some data on exposure of workers at sewage treatment facilities and at indoor pools and spas have also been reported. Lurker et al. (1983) reported a maximum level of 0.02 mg/m^3 in sewage treatment facilities. Maintenance workers, attendants and life guards at indoor pools and spas were exposed to 0.025 and 0.075 mg/m^3, respectively (Armstrong & Golden, 1986; Benoit & Jackson, 1987).

Generally low levels of chloroform were detected by Rosenberg et al. (1991) in a softwood and hardwood kraft pulp mill. Chloroform levels ranged from 50 to 290 μg/m^3 and from 220 to 5400 μg/m^3 in the softwood and the hardwood bleaching plants, respectively.

Chloroform has been and still is often used in dentistry as one of the ingredients of root canal sealers or as a solvent. The results of a study by Allard & Andersson (1992) showed that a dental team could be exposed to quite high concentrations, ranging from 2.2 to 19.1 mg/m^3.

6. KINETICS IN LABORATORY ANIMALS AND HUMANS

6.1 Pharmacokinetics

6.1.1 Absorption

6.1.1.1 Oral

Chloroform is well absorbed after oral administration. After intragastric administration of chloroform (75 mg/kg body weight) in water or vegetable oil to male Wistar rats, peak blood concentrations were observed in about 6 min, but blood concentrations were higher (39.3 versus 5.9 μg/ml) with water than with olive oil as the vehicle (Withey et al., 1983). The area under the blood concentration-time course curve (AUC) after chloroform administration in water was 8.7 times greater than the AUC derived from vegetable oil delivery.

Corley et al. (1990) used the data of Withey et al. (1983) to compute gavage absorption rate constants, which were 0.6 h^{-1} and 5.0 h^{-1} for corn oil and water, respectively.

6.1.1.2 Dermal

Chloroform is absorbed through the intact skin. Most studies have examined the systemic appearance of chloroform (or its appearance in expired air) to quantify absorption. Tsuruta (1975) estimated an absorption rate of 329 nmol/min per cm^2 of skin surface for pure chloroform in mice, but this study did not correct for metabolism. Morgan et al. (1991) measured blood chloroform levels in male F-344 rats during 24-h dermal exposures of a shaved region of the back to pure chloroform or to aqueous chloroform solutions. The blood chloroform level peaked at 51 mg/litre after exposure to the pure chemical for 4 to 8 h, and remained about constant for the duration of the exposure period. More rapid absorption rates were observed during exposure to the aqueous solutions, which resulted in peak blood chloroform levels after about 2 h. The authors attributed this difference to hydration of the skin. Bogen et al. (1992) applied aqueous solutions of [^{14}C]-chloroform to most of the body surface of hairless guinea-pigs and obtained a permeability coefficient of 0.13 ml/cm^2 per h. This study recovered metabolites as well as expired chloroform to measure absorption.

Indirect evidence of chloroform absorption was obtained by observation of damage to kidney tubules in rabbits treated with 1, 2 or 4 g chloroform/kg applied under an impermeable plastic cuff held tightly to the belly of rabbits for 24 h (Torkelson et al., 1976).

3.1.1.3 Inhalation

Lehmann & Hasegawa (1910) exposed rabbits to chloroform vapour concentrations of around 20, 54 or 80 g/m³. About 35% of the inhaled dose was retained during the first hour of the exposure period. The fraction retained declined progressively after longer periods of exposure (5 to 10% after 4 h; 2% after 8 h). In dogs exposed to 73.2 g chloroform/m³, a steady-state blood concentration of 354 mg chloroform/litre was reached within 2 h (Von Oettingen et al., 1950).

Corley et al. (1990) developed a pharmacokinetic model for chloroform (see section 6.1.4), which was based on inhalation studies in a closed-atmosphere chamber (concentrations of 490-24 500 mg/m³; 100-5000 ppm). Given the same chloroform concentration (4900 mg/m³; 1000 ppm), uptake over 6 h in male B6C3F$_1$ mice (total body weight = 450 g) was much more rapid and complete than in male F-344 rats (total body weight = 690 g). This difference is due primarily to the higher rate of chloroform metabolism in mice.

6.1.2 Distribution

Cohen & Hood (1969) performed autoradiography studies in male NMRI mice after inhalation or intravenous injection of anaesthetic doses of chloroform and found high levels of radioactivity in fat and liver. Following a 10-min inhalation exposure, the tissue:blood ratios at 0, 15 and 120 min post-exposure were 1.56, 2.10 and 6.7 for the liver and 6.42, 9.25 and 7.18 for fat, respectively. The increase in radioactivity in the liver was attributed to the accumulation of non-volatile, ether-extractable products. Other tissues (blood, brain, muscle, lung and kidney) contained lesser and more uniform amounts of radioactivity. Two hours after intravenous injection of [14C]-chloroform, non-volitive radioactivity in the liver accounted for 2% of the total dose.

Bergman (1984) studied the distribution of [14C]-chloroform in mice after inhalation of 5 μl of [14C]-chloroform (reported dose: 280 mg/kg) during 10 min. Whole-body autoradiography, immediately after exposure and 2 h thereafter, showed high concentrations of radioactivity in fat, blood, lungs, liver, kidneys, spinal cord and nerves, meninges and cerebellar cortex. After heating and extraction of the sections, it appeared that non-volatile radioactivity was bound in the bronchi, nasal mucosa, liver, kidneys, salivary glands and in the duodenal contents. High levels of volatile or extractable radioactivity were found in testes, preputial gland and epididymis.

Danielsson et al. (1986) observed tissue binding in gestational C57BL mice and their fetuses after inhalation of very low concentrations of [^{14}C]-chloroform for 10 min, and in 4-day-old C57BL mice after intraperitoneal injection of 0.4 μmoles of [^{14}C]-chloroform, respectively. The animals were killed 0, 1, 4 and 24 h after exposure. Low temperature autoradiograms, as well as scintillation spectrometry, showed a high uptake of radioactivity (volatile and non-volatile) directly after inhalation, especially in the respiratory epithelium and liver, fat, lung, brain and segments of tubuli in the renal cortex. Tissue-bound (non-volatile) radioactivity was found in the respiratory tract, centrilobular regions of the liver, salivary glands, and the conjunctiva of the eye. Volatile radioactivity was no longer present 24 h after exposure and the non-volatile activity had decreased with time in all organs measured. Accumulation of non-volatile metabolites was also found in the fetal respiratory tract.

The placental transport of chloroform was first demonstrated by Nicloux (1906) in guinea-pigs. Danielsson et al. (1986) reported that chloroform was transported to the conceptus at all stages of gestation in mice. Non-volatile metabolites of chloroform accumulated in the conceptus with time, especially in the amniotic fluid at mid-gestation. The fetal uptake of chloroform was low, which, according to the authors, was attributable to the low fat content in the fetus. An accumulation of non-extractable metabolites was found in the fetal respiratory tract in late gestation.

Withey & Karpinski (1985) exposed Sprague-Dawley rats on the 17th day of pregnancy to a series of different concentrations of chloroform (111 to 1984 ppm; 544 to 9722 mg/m^3) for 5 h. Chloroform distribution did not appear to be related to fetal position in the uterine horn. There was a highly significant inter-litter variation in fetal concentration, and additional tests showed that the maternal chloroform concentration accounted for only part of the variation. However, the fetal and maternal blood concentrations were linear functions of the administered dose, with a fetal/maternal ratio of 0.316.

A sex difference in tissue-bound radioactivity in mice given [^{14}C]-chloroform was reported by Taylor et al. (1974). Autoradiographic studies showed that the renal cortex of male CF/LP, CBA and C57BL mice accumulated more label than the renal cortex of female mice of the same strains. Treatment with testosterone resulted in an increase in tissue binding in the females and castration reduced the binding in the males (Taylor et al., 1974). Sex differences in renal binding were not found in the rat or monkey (Brown et al., 1974b).

6.1.3 Elimination and fate

The results of a pharmacokinetic study in male Wistar rats indicated that the elimination of chloroform after intravenous administration (jugular vein) at dose levels of 3, 6, 9, 12 or 15 mg/kg body weight followed a three-compartment model. Chloroform was eliminated at a slower rate from fat (half-life of 106 min) than from any other tissue examined. The elimination rates from all tissues, except fat, were similar to those derived from blood analysis (Whithey & Collins, 1980). The elimination half-lives for the water and vegetable oil vehicles were 46 and 39 min, respectively.

Various studies on the elimination of chloroform have been reported (Paul & Rubinstein, 1963; Van Dyke et al., 1964; Lavigne & Marchand, 1974). Corley et al. (1990) exposed B6C3F$_1$ mice and Osborne-Mendel rats to a range of chloroform concentrations for 6 h and measured the radioactivity in exhaled air, urine, faeces, carcass and skin and in the cage wash (Table 6). The fraction of the dose exhaled as unchanged chloroform increased with increasing exposure concentration in both mice and rats. [^{14}C]-CO$_2$ was the major metabolite exhaled. The data indicate partial metabolic saturation at the higher doses studied.

Brown et al. (1974b) administered [^{14}C]-chloroform (60 mg/kg body weight) to mice, rats and squirrel monkeys by the oral route. The radioactivity was measured in the exhaled air, urine, faeces and carcasses up to 48 h after dosing. The recovery percentages (of the dose) are listed in Table 7.

About 50% of the radioactivity in the urine of the mouse and the rat consisted of [^{14}C]-urea and [^{14}C]-bicarbonate. Autoradiography revealed biliary excretion of radioactivity in the monkey. A high concentration of radioactivity in the bile was present as unchanged chloroform.

Table 6. Radioactivity (mg eq/kg body weight) in B6C3F$_1$ mice and
Osborne-Mendel rats during and up to 48 h after 6-h exposures to
[^{14}C]-chloroform (From: Corley et al., 1990)

Concen-tration (ppm)	Exhaled ^{14}C-chloroform	Exhaled ^{14}C-CO$_2$	Urine	Faeces	Residue[a]
Mice					
10	0.03	7.22	0.95	0.05	0.19
89	0.47	70.35	7.46	1.24	2.32
366	23.03	217.85	21.24	3.84	9.68
Rats					
93	0.76	31.84	3.34	0.40	1.09
356	16.15	54.85	6.53	0.81	2.18
1041	78.27	89.04	11.83	1.16	3.95

[a]   Residues comprising total ^{14}C-label present in carcass, skin and cage wash at the
end of post-exposure collection period

Table 7. Percentage recovery of radioactivity after [^{14}C]-chloroform
administration (From: Brown et al., 1974b)

Species	In breath		In faeces and urine	In carcass[a]
	chloroform	CO$_2$		
Mouse	5.2-7.1	84-87	2.1-3.0	1.2-2.3
Rat	20	67	8	NA
Monkey	79	18	2	NA

[a]   NA = not analysed

The excreted quantities of chloroform and carbon dioxide in
the rat, as reported by Brown et al. (1974b), correspond to those
reported by Reynolds et al. (1984), who found that after oral doses

of 12 or 36 mg chloroform/kg body weight to the rat, about 70% of the dose was excreted as carbon dioxide and 12% as chloroform in the 24 h following oral administration.

6.1.4 Physiologically based pharmacokinetic modelling for chloroform

Corley et al. (1990) developed a physiologically based pharmacokinetic model (PBPK) for mice, rats and humans that incorporated literature values for physiological parameters, tissue partition coefficients and metabolic constants. The metabolic constants were derived from results of rodent *in vivo* gas-uptake studies and *in vitro* metabolic studies with rodent and human (n=9) microsomes. The tissue:air partition coefficients were determined by a vial-equilibration technique with tissue homogenates. Macromolecular binding constants, which define the fraction of the total metabolites that bind covalently to proteins, were estimated from *in vivo* binding data obtained following inhalation exposures to radiolabelled chloroform. The model parameters that were derived for the three species by Corley et al. (1990) are presented in Table 8.

Table 8. Parameters used in the physiologically based pharmacokinetic model for chloroform[a]

	Mouse	Rat	Human
Partition coefficients			
Blood/air	21.3	20.8	7.43
Liver/air	19.1	21.1	17.0
Kidney/air	11.0	11.0	11.0
Fat/air	242	203	280
Rapidly perfused/air	19.1	21.1	17.0
Slowly perfused/air	13.0	13.9	12.0
Metabolic and macromolecular binding constants			
V_{maxC} (mg/h per kg)	22.8	6.8	15.7
K_m (mg/litre)	0.352	0.543	0.448
fMMB[b] (h^{-1}), liver	0.003	0.00104	0.00202
fMMB[b] (h^{-1}), kidney	0.010	0.0086	0.00931

[a]   From: Corley et al. (1990)
[b]   MMB = macromolecular binding of reactive metabolites; fMMB = fraction of MMB of particular organ

The blood:air partition coefficients for rodents were approximately three times greater than for humans. Metabolism was described by a single saturable pathway for each species, but in mice, equations accounting for enzyme loss had to be incorporated. The V_{maxC} values reflect the greater metabolic capacity of the mouse compared to the rat, which has been shown in numerous studies. The model generated predictions consistent with experimental data for target organ-specific protein binding in rodents as well as total chloroform metabolized and total exhaled chloroform in both rodents and humans. Predictions of protein binding suggest a relative sensitivity ranking for the three species as follows: mouse > rat > humans, assuming that equivalent levels of binding produce equivalent toxicities in target tissues (Corley et al., 1990).

Blancato & Chiu (1993) used the PBPK model of Corley et al. (1990) to predict the relative contributions of different exposure routes to target tissue doses of chloroform in humans. Tissue macromolecular binding was predicted as a dose surrogate. With respect to liver dose, a 10-min shower was predicted to contribute about 25% of the total dose, with 57% from drinking-water. Showering was predicted to account for more than 53% of the total dose to the kidney, while drinking-water was estimated to contribute only 7% of the dose. This difference was attributed to the absence of a first-pass effect with dermal absorption and inhalation exposures.

Gearhart et al. (1993) recently described an additional PBPK model for chloroform in B6C3F₁ mice. This model accounts for decreases in body temperature associated with exposure to high chloroform concentrations. The authors contend that the inclusion of an enzyme loss equation for mice in the model of Corley et al. (1990) was inappropriate and that the incorporation of temperature corrections greatly improved the overall fit of gas uptake data. The authors also obtained better model simulations of gas-uptake data by including a first-order rate constant, which is consistent with *in vitro* work demonstrating multiple pathways of chloroform biotransformation (Pohl, 1979; Testai et al., 1990).

6.2 Biotransformation and covalent binding of metabolites

Chloroform may undergo both oxidative and reductive biotransformation (Fig. 1). The oxygenation of chloroform is catalysed by cytochrome P450 and produces trichloromethanol. Elimination of HCl from trichloromethanol gives phosgene as a reactive intermediate (Mansuy et al., 1977; Pohl et al., 1977).

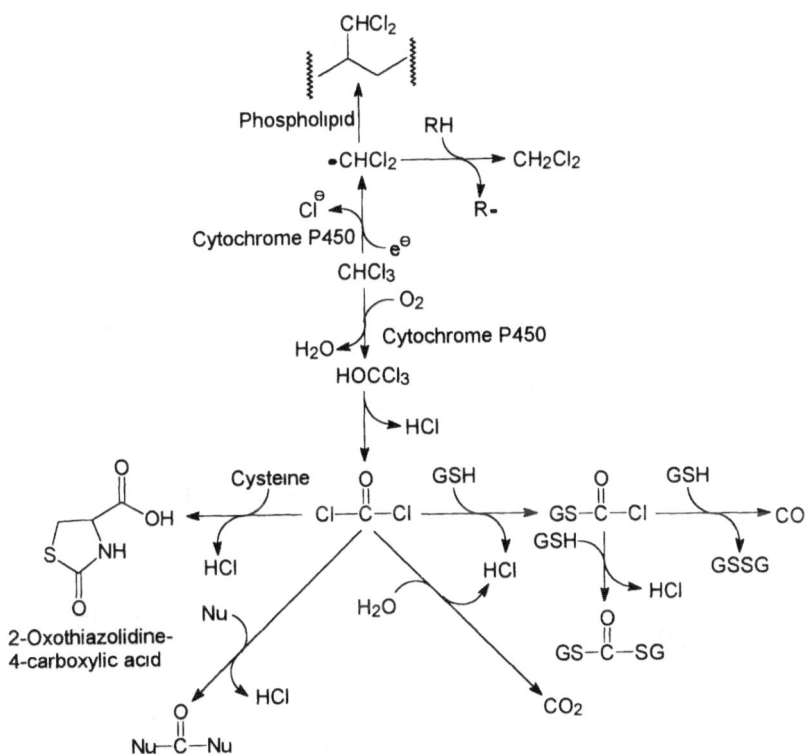

Fig. 1. Biotransformation of chloroform

There is considerable evidence available to support this reaction mechanism for the formation of phosgene in the biotransformation of chloroform: the biotransformation of chloroform to phosgene requires NADPH and oxygen. The phosgene formed in the biotransformation of chloroform can be trapped by reaction with cysteine to give 2-oxothiazolidine-4-carboxylic acid, and the biotransformation of [^{14}C]-chloroform in the presence of cysteine gives [^{14}C]-2-oxothiazolidine-4-carboxylic acid. When the biotransformation of chloroform was studied in the presence of [^{18}O]-dioxygen or [^{35}S]-cysteine, [2-^{18}O]- and [1-^{35}S]-2-oxothiazolidine-4-carboxylic acid, respectively, are formed. Deuterochloroform is biotransformed more slowly than chloroform (Mansuy et al., 1977; Pohl et al., 1977, 1979, 1980; Pohl & Krishna, 1978). Moreover, when [^{36}Cl]-chloroform, [^{3}H]-chloroform, or [^{14}C]-chloroform were incubated with liver microsomes from phenobarbital-treated Sprague-Dawley rats, only label from [^{14}C]-chloroform became covalently bound to proteins (Pohl et al., 1980).

Phosgene reacts rapidly with water to give CO_2 and HCl as products, which explains the formation of CO_2 as a metabolite of chloroform (Fry et al., 1972; Brown et al., 1974b). Phosgene may also react with tissue nucleophiles to form covalently bound products (Uehleke & Werner, 1975). Cysteine blocks the covalent binding of [^{14}C]-chloroform-derived radioactivity, which supports a role for phosgene in the formation of covalent adducts from chloroform (Pohl et al., 1977, 1980). Alternatively, phosgene may react with glutathione to form S-(chlorocarbonyl)glutathione; this intermediate may react with glutathione to give diglutathionyl dithiocarbonate (Pohl et al., 1981) or to give glutathione disulfide and carbon monoxide as minor products (Ahmed et al., 1977).

The reductive biotransformation of chloroform is also catalysed by cytochromes P450 (Testai & Vittozzi, 1986) (Fig. 1). Reduction of chloroform gives rise to the dichloromethyl radical, which has been identified by spin trapping and ESR (Tomasi et al., 1985). No evidence for the formation of the dichloromethyl carbanion has been presented, whereas the formation of chlorocarbene has been ruled out (Wolf et al., 1977). The dichloromethyl radical may react preferentially with the fatty acid skeleton of phospholipids to give covalently bound adducts (De Biasi et al., 1992).

The balance between the oxidative and reductive biotransformation of chloroform depends on several factors, including oxygen and chloroform concentrations, animal species, strain, enzyme induction, and the site of metabolism. Oxidative metabolism is favoured at low (< 0.1 mM) chloroform concentrations (Testai et al., 1990, 1991). Under these conditions, the oxygenation of chloroform is catalysed by cytochrome P450 2E1 (Brady et al., 1989; Guengerich et al., 1991), and covalent binding of chloroform metabolites to proteins and lipids in incubation mixtures containing mouse (B6C3F$_1$ or C57BL/6J) liver microsomes is higher than in incubation mixtures containing rat (Osborne-Mendel or Sprague-Dawley) liver microsomes (Testai et al., 1991).

Chloroform reduction is increased at high substrate concentrations (Testai et al., 1990), but oxidative metabolism is quantitatively more important. In incubation mixtures containing 5 mM chloroform, both oxygenation and reduction of chloroform depend on the oxygen tension in the incubation flask. Chloroform reduction is particularly evident with microsomes from B6C3F$_1$ mice and Osborne-Mendel rats. At high chloroform concentrations (~5 mM), the oxygenation of chloroform may be catalysed by cytochrome P450 2B1, as suggested by the induction of the metabolism due to pretreatment by phenobarbital (Branchflower et al., 1983; Testai & Vittozzi, 1986; Nakajima et al., 1991). Phenobarbital or β-naphthoflavone pretreatment of Sprague-Dawley rats also stimulates the formation of reduced intermediates of chloroform (Testai & Vittozzi, 1986). Levels of the *in vitro* covalent binding of [^{14}C]-chloroform metabolites to proteins were higher with hepatic microsomes from rabbits and human biopsies than with hepatic microsomes from rats or mice (Uehleke & Werner, 1975).

The *in vitro* formation of dichloromethane as a stable end-product of chloroform metabolism was addressed in early studies. Dichloromethane was detected in mouse liver slices incubated with chloroform (Butler, 1961), but not in slices or subcellular fractions of rat liver incubated with chloroform (Paul & Rubinstein, 1963; Rubinstein & Kanics, 1964). These discrepancies, however, may have been due to the incubation conditions employed in these early studies. *In vivo* results with rats, dogs, mice and human volunteers exposed to chloroform consistently indicated no expiration of dichloromethane (Butler, 1961; Paul & Rubinstein, 1963; Fry et al., 1972; Brown et al., 1974b).

Interspecies differences in the oxidative metabolism of chloroform have been found *in vivo*. After a [^{14}C]-chloroform dose of 60 mg/kg body weight, 85%, 66% and 18% was excreted as $[^{14}C]$-CO_2 in C57BL, CF/PL and CBA mice, Sprague-Dawley rats, and squirrel monkeys, respectively. Expiration of ^{14}C accounted for the elimination of most of the remaining dose (recoveries of 93-98%) (Brown et al., 1974b). Mink et al. (1986) and Corley et al. (1990) also showed that chloroform is metabolized in the mouse to a greater extent than in the rat. Corley et al. (1990) demonstrated that the covalent binding of $[^{14}C]$-chloroform metabolites to liver and kidney proteins *in vivo* was higher in B6C3F$_1$ mice than in Osborne-Mendel rats.

In several strains of mice given $[^{14}C]$-chloroform, more binding occurred in the kidney tissue of males than in that of females (Ilett et al., 1973; Taylor et al., 1974). Male DBA mice accumulate twice as much radioactivity in their kidneys as do male C57BL mice. This strain difference shows intermediate or multifactorial heredity (Hill et al., 1975).

Differences in binding were associated with variations in toxicity (Hill et al., 1975; Clemens et al., 1979). The nephrotoxicity of chloroform in male mice of susceptible strains (see chapter 7) is most probably related to *in situ* renal metabolic activation of chloroform (Zaleska-Rutczynska & Krus, 1973; Hill, 1978; Clemens et al., 1979; Smith & Hook, 1983; Smith et al., 1984). Indeed the overall biotransformation of chloroform in both sexes is equal, whereas males exhibit more extensive formation of renal tissue-bound metabolites than females (Taylor et al., 1974; Smith & Hook, 1984). Smith et al. (1985) observed little chloroform metabolism in rat (male, Fischer-344) renal cortical microsomes. Additional studies, however, have demonstrated chloroform-induced cytolethality and regenerative cell damage in male, Fischer-344 rat kidney (Larson et al., 1993). Culliford & Hewitt (1957) reported that females became more susceptible after pretreatment with androgens, and the sensitivity of the males was reduced after castration.

In the rat and mouse, chloroform biotransformation occurs mainly in the liver, but other tissues also show metabolic activity. After oral administration of chloroform to mice, maximum covalent binding in the liver was observed after 3 h, whereas in the kidney, maximum binding was found after 6 to 12 h. Binding appears to be dose dependent up to doses of 3 mmol/kg body weight. At higher doses, a plateau is reached (Ilett et al., 1973). Löfberg & Tjälve (1986) studied the extra-hepatic metabolism of $[^{14}C]$-chloroform in Sprague-Dawley rats. Autoradiography was used to localize metabolites in freeze-dried, extracted tissues to distinguish between total and bound radioactivity. *In vitro* autoradiography, in which tissue slices were incubated with [^{14}C]-chloroform and then examined autoradiographically, showed the capacity of several tissues to metabolize [^{14}C]-chloroform: liver, kidney cortex, mucosa of the bronchial tree, tracheal mucosa, olfactory and respiratory nasal mucosa, Bowman's glands in the olfactory lamina propria mucosae, Steno's gland (the lateral nasal gland), mucosa of the oesophagus, larynx, tongue, gingiva, cheek, naso-pharyngeal duct, pharynx and the soft palate. Furthermore, autoradiographic studies showed that a correlation exists between the ability of the tissues to retain metabolites *in vivo* and the ability of these tissues to metabolize chloroform *in vitro*.

The distribution of the covalent binding of ^{14}C to DNA or RNA after an intraperitoneal injection of [^{14}C]-chloroform to Balb/c mice or to Wistar rats shows several differences from the distribution of the covalent binding to tissue proteins (Colacci et al., 1991). The highest levels of covalent binding to DNA were observed in mouse kidney (3.17 nmol/g DNA) and lung (3.65 nmol/g DNA). In mice, binding to liver DNA (0.83 nmol/g DNA) was lower than binding to stomach DNA (1.52 nmol/g DNA).

Differences in DNA binding of chloroform metabolites among rat organs have been found to be limited, and the absolute values were lower than those seen in mouse organs. In mice, RNA binding levels were high in both the liver and kidney; in rats, they were higher in the kidney than in other organs. In mice, protein binding was highest in the liver (47.5 nmol/g), whereas in rats it was high in both the liver (27.4 nmol/g) and kidney (30.7 nmol/g). In incubations containing low (< 0.1 mM) chloroform concentrations and human liver microsomes, little formation of reactive metabolites was seen (Vittozzi et al., 1991). Detectable covalent binding was observed in microsomes from some samples of colonic and ileal mucosa of human patients but not of male Sprague-Dawley rats (Testai et al., 1991).

Glutathione (GSH) is an important factor controlling the binding of chloroform metabolites to proteins and lipids. In *in vitro* studies, physiological concentrations of GSH (2-5 mM) strongly reduced the covalent binding of chloroform metabolites to proteins (Sipes et al., 1977; Cresteil et al., 1979; Smith & Hook, 1984). In later studies, 3 mM GSH blocked the covalent binding of chloroform metabolites to proteins and to phospholipid polar heads, whereas covalent binding to the phospholipid fatty acyl chains (due to the radical metabolite) was only slightly affected

(Testai & Vittozzi, 1986; Testai et al., 1990, 1991; De Biasi et al., 1992). Pretreatment of rats with diethylmaleate or buthionine sulfoximine (BSO) increased the binding of administered [^{14}C]-chloroform to proteins (Stevens & Anders, 1981). Pretreatment of phenobarbital-induced Sprague-Dawley rats with cysteine decreased the covalent binding (Stevens & Anders, 1981b). Toxic effects paralleled the covalent binding levels after these pretreatments (Stevens & Anders, 1981a).

6.3 Human studies

6.3.1 Uptake

6.3.1.1 Oral

When Fry et al. (1972) dosed eight volunteers with 0.5 g chloroform in olive oil in capsules, approximately 50% of the oral dose was metabolized to carbon dioxide. Maximal blood levels of 1 to 5 ng chloroform/litre were achieved after 1.5 h. In two of the subjects, the decline in blood levels could be described by a two-compartment model with a half-life of 13 min for the initial phase and a half-life of 90 min for the second phase. Chiou (1975) reanalysed the data obtained from the two subjects mentioned above and calculated an apparent volume of distribution of approximately 160 litres. The author estimated the hepatic first-pass effect to be about 32% and the pulmonary first-pass effect to be 16%. Hence after a single oral dose of 0.5 g chloroform, about 52% of the dose may be available to the system. Pulmonary and metabolic clearances of 0.7 and 0.6 litre/min, respectively, gave a total body clearance of 1.3 litre/min.

6.3.1.2 Dermal

Jo et al. (1990a) studied the relative contributions of dermal and pulmonary uptake of chloroform in individuals taking showers. Post-exposure exhaled air concentrations of chloroform were measured to estimate chloroform uptake and were 6 to 21 $\mu g/m^3$ for normal showers and 2.4 to 10 $\mu g/m^3$ for inhalation-only exposure. The difference between normal and inhalation-only exposure was significant, and the authors concluded that the contribution of dermal exposure was approximately equivalent to inhalation exposure.

Chinery & Gleason (1993) modified an existing PBPK model to predict the exhaled air concentration of chloroform in individuals exposed to the chemical while showering. Calibration of the model with measured exhaled air concentrations of chloroform in individuals exposed while showering either with or without dermal absorption generated an expected value for skin-blood partitioning of 1.2. This assumes a degree of transfer of chloroform from shower water into shower air of 61%. The stratum corneum permeability coefficient for chloroform was estimated to be within a range of 0.16-0.36 cm/h, and the expected value was 0.2 cm/h. The estimated ratio of dermally:inhaled absorbed doses while showering ranged between 0.6 and 2.2 and the expected value was 0.75.

6.3.1.3 Inhalation

The inhalation uptake of chloroform in humans was studied by Lehmann & Hasegawa in 1910. More recently, Morgan et al. (1970) measured the absorption of chloroform after a single inhalation exposure to approximately 5 mg of [^{38}Cl]-chloroform. About 80% of the chloroform was absorbed under these conditions.

Prolonged inhalation of anaesthetic concentrations (about 50 g chloroform/m^3 air) gave rise to blood chloroform concentrations of about 100 mg/litre (Smith et al., 1973).

The relative contribution of inhalation to chloroform uptake during showering has been determined (see section 6.3.1.2, Jo et al., 1990a).

6.3.2 Distribution

Corley et al. (1990) determined partition coefficients for human tissues (see Table 8).

McConnell et al. (1975) analysed chloroform levels in postmortem tissue from eight persons (four males and four females, 48 to 82 years old) living in non-industrial areas of the United Kingdom. The chloroform levels (μg/kg wet tissue weight) observed were: body fat, 5-68 (mean = 51); liver, 1-10 (mean = 7.2); kidney, 2-5; and brain, 2-4.

Phillips & Birchard (1991) reported on a nationwide survey of the general population by the US EPA's National Human Adipose Tissue Survey. Several hundred fat samples were pooled into 46 composite samples by age and geographic region and were analysed. Chloroform was detected at levels ranging from 5 to 580 ng/g in 29 of the composite samples.

Dowty et al. (1976) detected chloroform in human maternal and placental cord blood. Erickson et al. (1981) found chloroform, supposedly originating from environmental exposure, present in mother's milk (concentration not specified). Chloroform was identified, but not quantified, in mother's milk samples collected from 49 lactating women living in the vicinity of chemical manufacturing plants or industrial user facilities in Pennsylvania, New Jersey and Louisiana, USA (Pellizzari et al., 1982).

6.3.3 Elimination

Human volunteers given oral doses of 500 mg chloroform eliminated on average 50% of the dose as CO_2 and 40% as unchanged chloroform during 8 h after dosing (Fry et al., 1972). The amount of expired chloroform varied from 18 to 66%, depending on the obesity of individuals.

After administration of 100, 250 or 1000 mg, the authors recovered 0, 12 and 65% of the dose in the expired air, respectively. After administration of [^{14}C]-chloroform to a man and a woman, approximately 50% of the dose was found in the exhaled air (as CO_2) in 7.5 h after dosing. Virtually no chloroform was excreted by the kidneys (Fry et al., 1972).

After inhalation of chloroform (concentrations of 21 or 35 g chloroform/m^3), Lehmann & Hasegawa (1910) found little pulmonary excretion, i.e. approximately 2% of the absorbed quantity within 30 min after the exposure. A pulmonary excretion of 10% of the body content during the first hour after exposure was reported by Morgan et al. (1970).

6.3.4 Biotransformation

Human cytochrome P450 2E1 catalyses the oxygenation of chloroform (Guengerich et al., 1991).

Corley et al. (1990) quantified CO_2 production from incubations of human liver microsomes with 0.049-0.058 mM chloroform. The average activity of samples from nine individuals was 8.15 ± 0.02 pmol chloroform oxidized/min per mg protein. These data were correlated with rodent *in vitro* and *in vivo* conversion rates to estimate human *in vivo* metabolic rate constants (see Table 8).

7. EFFECTS ON LABORATORY MAMMALS AND *IN VITRO* TEST SYSTEMS

7.1 Single exposure

7.1.1 Lethality

The LD_{50} values of chloroform for mice and rats are given in Tables 9 and 10, respectively. Chloroform-induced death is usually due to liver damage, with the exception of male mice of very sensitive strains, whose death is caused by kidney damage. The higher susceptibility to chloroform acute toxicity in these strains of mice (such as DBA, C3H, C3Hf, CBA, Balb/c, C3H/He), with respect to other strains, is genetically controlled. An absolute sex-related difference with respect to kidney damage, but not to liver damage, has been described in mice: female mice do not develop renal lesions. This is independent of the strain. Some influence of age on chloroform acute toxicity in rats has also been described (Kimura et al., 1971).

For the rat, the LD_{50} values ranged from 450 to 2000 mg chloroform/kg body weight, and in this species no sex difference in susceptibility was found (Kimura et al., 1971; Chu et al., 1980). For OF1 female mice, a LC_{50} value of 6150 mg chloroform/m^3 (6 h exposure) was reported by Gradiski et al. (1978).

A dose of 3070 mg chloroform/kg body weight in mineral oil to rats resulted in death due to CNS depression within minutes, and a dose of 980 mg chloroform/kg body weight resulted in hepatic centrilobular necrosis (Reynolds & Yee, 1967). When administered to newborn rats, chloroform was lethal at oral doses of 1500 mg/kg body weight; smaller doses were not administered (Kimura et al., 1971).

7.1.2 Non-lethal effects

1.2.1 Oral exposure

Chloroform is a potent anaesthetic. Anaesthesia may result from oral administration of chloroform; this was established by Bowman et al. (1978) in the ICR mouse with a dose of 500 mg chloroform/kg body weight in aqueous emulsion. The ED_{50} (50% of animals showing effect at this dose level) in mice for acute neurological effects (ataxia, incoordination and anaesthesia) was 484 mg chloroform/kg body weight (Balster & Borzelleca, 1982).

Table 9. Representative LD_{50} values (mg chloroform/kg body weight) for mice

Sex/strain	Route	Vehicle	Observed period	LD_{50}	Reference
Male					
C3H/tif	oral	sesame oil	15 days	36	Pericin & Thomann (1979)
DBA/2/j	oral	sesame oil	15 days	101	Pericin & Thomann (1979)
Tif:MAGf	oral	sesame oil	15 days	213	Pericin & Thomann (1979)
A/J	oral	sesame oil	15 days	253	Pericin & Thomann (1979)
Tif:MF2f	oral	sesame oil	15 days	336	Pericin & Thomann (1979)
C57BL/6J	oral	sesame oil	15 days	460	Pericin & Thomann (1979)
Princeton	subcutaneous	peanut oil	10 days	696	Plaa et al. (1958)
Swiss albino	subcutaneous	olive oil	10 days	3245	Kutob & Plaa (1962a)
Female					
C3H/tif	oral	sesame oil	15 days	353	Pericin & Thomann (1979)
DBA/2/j	oral	sesame oil	15 days	679	Pericin & Thomann (1979)
A/J	oral	sesame oil	15 days	774	Pericin & Thomann (1979)
C57BL/6J	oral	sesame oil	15 days	820	Pericin & Thomann (1979)
Tif:MF2f	oral	sesame oil	15 days	1126	Pericin & Thomann (1979)
Tif:MAGf	oral	sesame oil	15 days	1366	Pericin & Thomann (1979)
OF1	intraperitoneal	olive oil	14 days	880	Gradiski et al. (1974)

Table 10. Representative LD$_{50}$ values (mg chloroform/kg body weight) for rats

Sex/strain	Route	Vehicle	Observed period	LD$_{50}$	Reference
Male					
Sprague-Dawley (14 days old)	oral	none	unknown	450	Kimura et al. (1971)
unknown (older adults)	oral	none	unknown	1200	Kimura et al. (1971)
Sprague-Dawaley	oral	none	14 days	908	Chu et al. (1980)
Sprague-Dawley	oral	none	14 days	2000	Torkelson et al. (1976)
Female					
Sprague-Dawley (14 days old)	oral	none	unknown	450	Kimura et al. (1971)
Sprague-Dawley	oral	none	14 days	1117	Chu et al. (1980)
Sprague-Dawley	intraperitoneal	peanut oil	24 h 14 days	1379 894	Lundberg et al. (1986)

65

After oral administration of chloroform in olive oil to Swiss mice (both sexes), Jones et al. (1958) found the median narcotic dose to be 350 mg/kg body weight and the median hepatotoxic dose to be 35 mg/kg body weight. At this dose level, the liver showed centrilobular fatty infiltration and at 350 mg/kg body weight centrilobular necrosis was found.

Hill (1978) investigated strain and sex differences in chloroform-induced toxicity in mice. Male mice of three strains (DBA/2J, B6D2F$_1$/J, and C57BL/6J) were given single oral doses of chloroform in oil. No clear difference in hepatotoxicity between strains was observed; centrilobular necrosis occurred at doses greater than 250 mg/kg body weight in all three strains. In contrast, there were differences between species in renal toxicity. Doses of 89 mg/kg body weight caused glucosuria and/or proteinuria in half of the DBA/2J animals, while doses of 119 and 163 mg/kg body weight were required to produce these effects in half the B6D2F$_1$/J and C57BL/6J mice, respectively.

In male CFLP Swiss mice, Moore et al. (1982) found neither histological changes in the liver or kidney nor biochemical changes in plasma 4 days after oral administration of 17 mg chloroform/kg body weight in corn oil. Administration of 66 mg chloroform/kg body weight caused slight hepatotoxicity and a more severe nephrotoxicity.

Chu et al. (1980, 1982a) observed piloerection, sedation, flaccid muscle tone, ataxia, prostration and dacryorrhoea after administration of chloroform to rats. Food intake in the males was reduced. Histological and biochemical examination revealed effects on liver, kidneys and red and white blood cells. Upon histological examination, no lesions were found in other tissues with chloroform doses up to 2100 mg/kg body weight. In this study the lowest administered dose was 546 mg chloroform/kg body weight, a level at which toxic effects were still found.

Reitz et al. (1982) determined the cellular regeneration (as ^{3}H-thymidine uptake in DNA) 48 h after administration of chloroform to male B6C3F$_1$ mice and male Osborne-Mendel rats. In the mice, ^{3}H-thymidine uptake was significantly increased in kidneys at a dose level of 60 mg chloroform/kg body weight and in kidneys and liver at 240 mg chloroform/kg body weight. In the rats, only a slight increase in ^{3}H-thymidine uptake in liver and kidneys was found at a dose level of 180 mg chloroform/kg body weight.

Torkelson et al. (1976) reported dose-related liver and kidney changes in adult rats at dose levels as low as 250 mg chloroform/kg body weight. Tyson et al. (1983) found an elevation of serum aminotransferase levels in rats at dose levels above 200 mg/kg body weight in oil.

One study examined the organ-specific toxicity of acute doses of chloroform (Larson et al., 1993). Male F-344 rats were given chloroform by gavage in corn oil at doses of 0, 34, 180 or 477 mg/kg body weight and necropsied 24 h later. Additional rats were given a single dose of 180 mg chloroform/kg and administered bromodeoxyuridine (BrdU) 2 h prior to necropsy at 0.5, 1, 2, 4, and 8 days after chloroform treatment to label cells in S-phase. The kidneys of male rats administered 34, 180 and 477 mg chloroform/kg exhibited mild to severe proximal tubular necrosis in a dose-dependent manner. A 20-fold increase in the labelling index (LI, % of nuclei in S-phase) in the proximal tubule cells was observed 2 days after treatment at a dose of 180 mg/kg body weight. The livers of the male rats exhibited only slight to moderate multifocal centrilobular necrosis at 180 and 477 mg/kg body weight. A 10-fold increase in the LI was observed in the liver of male rats given 477 mg/kg body weight, but no increase was observed at 180 mg/kg body weight (Larson et al., 1993).

Female $B6C3F_1$ mice were given chloroform by gavage (0, 34, 238 or 477 mg/kg body weight) and necropsied 24 h after treatment. Additional mice were given a single dose of 350 mg chloroform/kg body weight, labelled with BrdU, and necropsied 0.5, 1, 2, 4, and 8 days after treatment. Female mice developed a dose-dependent centrilobular hepatic necrosis at 238 and 477 mg/kg body weight. No renal lesions were observed in female mice at any dose. A peak increase in LI of 38-fold was observed in hepatocytes in the livers of female mice 2 days after treatment with 350 mg chloroform/kg, but the increase in LI observed in the kidneys was only 2-fold (Larson et al., 1993). These data indicate that acute chloroform-induced cytolethality leads to increased cell proliferation and that the organ-specific pattern of toxicity is the same as the organ-specific pattern of tumour formation (see NCI, 1976a,b, and section 7.7.1).

Groger & Grey (1979) intubated Colworth Wistar rats (6 of each sex per group) daily with chloroform in peanut oil (0 to 50 mg/kg body weight) for periods of 1, 5 or 10 days. There were changes in the activity of several liver enzymes, the toxicological significance of which is unclear.

Balster & Borzelleca (1982) administered chloroform in water to male ICR mice (8-12/group) and examined their performances in a battery of neurobehavioural tests (several exposure periods and several dose levels). The only effect observed was a reduced achievement in an operant behaviour test after dosing with 100 and 400 mg chloroform/kg body weight in water for 60 days. At the chloroform level of 400 mg/kg body weight, about half the treated animals died. No adverse effects on behaviour were observed after 90 days of dosing with 31 mg chloroform/kg body weight in water.

7.1.2.2 Subcutaneous and intraperitoneal exposure

A sex difference in toxicity was found after subcutaneous and intraperitoneal administration of chloroform to mice. In males, the kidney appeared to be more susceptible than in females, in which the liver was found to be the target organ. Smith et al. (1983) exposed male and female mice of the ICR strain to chloroform doses of 75 to 1500 mg/kg body weight (subcutaneous and intraperitoneal). Hepatotoxicity was dose-related in both sexes from 375 mg chloroform/kg body weight upwards. After the subcutaneous administration of 375 mg chloroform/kg body weight, an increase in the serum alanine aminotransferase (ALAT) and a decrease in the liver non-protein sulfhydryl groups (NPSH) were observed. Histological examinations showed centrilobular swelling of the liver and necrosis of the hepatocytes in both sexes. At 24 h after intraperitoneal exposure to 375 mg chloroform/kg body weight, renal toxicity was observed in males but not in females. A decrease in the renal NPSH concentration of about 60% in males and 20% in females was found. The concentration in females, but not in males, returned to normal within 24 h post-dosing. Histological examination of male kidneys showed proximal tubular lesions with pyknotic nuclei and loss of reticular cytoplasmic structure, necrosis of the cells of the proximal tubuli and occlusion of the tubular lumens with hyaline casts (Smith et al., 1983).

Skrzypinska et al. (1991) administered chloroform intraperitoneally to Balb/c mice as a single dose ranging from 12.5 to 100% of the approximate lethal dose. At different time periods after administration, mice were sacrificed. Serum glutamine-pyruvate transaminase (SGPT) and sorbitol dehydrogenase (SDH), as well as glutathione (GSH) and malondialdehyde (MDA) levels in the liver, were determined. Increased SGPT and SDH levels were found for all doses exceeding one eighth of the approximate lethal dose. The depletion of GSH level was kept within 40% for all doses. A 2- to 4-fold increase of hepatic MDA level was found. The depletion of hepatic GSH, and to some extent the increase of SGPT and SDH, occurred in a biphasic fashion. Dose-effect functions for these biochemical alterations could only be constructed for the second delayed phase of action. It is postulated that the hepatotoxicity of chloroform is mainly dependent on radical formation in the course of biotransformation.

Plaa & Larson (1965) observed renal toxicity after an intraperitoneal dose as low as 48 mg chloroform/kg body weight in male Swiss mice. The authors reported that chloroform was the most potent nephrotoxic agent of 14 short-chain chlorinated hydrocarbons in male mice.

Ahmadizadeh et al. (1984) found an increase in the relative kidney weight after intraperitoneal administration of chloroform in peanut oil (150 mg/kg body weight) to male DBA mice, but not after chloroform administration to DBA female mice or to male or female mice of the C57BL strain.

Hepatic toxicity, which is the predominant effect in most species, was found after a parenteral dose of 450 and 150 mg chloroform/kg body weight in the rat and the guinea-pig, respectively (Klaassen & Plaa, 1969; Divincenzo & Krasavage, 1974).

Detection of lipoperoxidation in the liver of PB-induced rats exposed to chloroform has been reported by several authors (Klaassen & Plaa, 1969; Brown, 1972; Brown et al., 1974a; Masuda et al., 1980).

An increased bile duct/pancreatic fluid flow and a changed composition of this fluid were observed after an intraperitoneal dose of 1500 mg chloroform/kg body weight to rats (Harms et al., 1976; Hamada & Peterson, 1977).

A single, liver-damaging intraperitoneal dose of chloroform led to a maximal glutathione depletion in the liver of PB-pretreated rats shortly after dosing (1-2 h) but not in saline-treated rats. However, the maximal histopathological findings (centrilobular necrosis) occurred much later (after about 24 h) (Docks & Krishna, 1976).

In dogs, liver toxicity has been found after intraperitoneal administration of chloroform. The ED_{50} for an increased serum ALAT activity via this route appears to be 300 mg chloroform/kg body weight. At near-ED_{50} doses, chloroform caused centrilobular vacuolization and centrilobular and subcapsular necrosis. The ED_{50} for renal dysfunction in the dog appears to be 645 mg chloroform/kg body weight (Klaassen & Plaa, 1967).

Bai et al. (1992) evaluated the suitability of nine different serum bile acids (SBA) as markers of chloroform exposure in rats. Increases in specific SBA levels were observed following three daily intraperitoneal administrations of chloroform at doses as low as 0.1 mmol/kg body weight. The effects on SBA levels were detectable at much lower doses than were effects on histopathological indices or on levels of alanine aminotransferase, aspartatetransaminase, alkaline phosphatase, bilirubin or total bile acid.

Chloroform doses as low as 45 mg/kg body weight reduced the microsomal Ca^{++}/Mg^{++}-ATP-ase activity (liver microsome calcium pump) in rats (Moore, 1980).

7.1.2.3 Inhalation exposure

After exposure to chloroform vapour, the same pattern of toxicity in mice was observed as after oral, intraperitoneal or subcutaneous administration (Deringer et al., 1953; Hewitt, 1956). Deringer et al. (1953) found necrosis in the proximal and distal convoluted tubules, hyaline casts in the convoluted tubules and collecting ducts, calcification of the cortex, and death after exposure of male C3H mice to chloroform concentrations of 3400 to 5400 mg/m³ for 1 to 3 h; anaesthesia was not observed.

Kylin et al. (1963) exposed female albino mice of an undefined strain to chloroform vapour for 4 h and reported hepatotoxic effects. At 24 h after exposure to chloroform concentrations of 490 mg/m³ or more, a concentration-related fatty infiltration was observed. From 980 mg chloroform/m³ upwards, necrosis of liver cells and a rise in the serum ornithine carbamoyltransferase level were seen. In mice, rabbits, guinea-pigs and cats, anaesthesia was induced by exposure to chloroform concentrations in the range of 10 to 100 g/m³ for periods of 30 min to a few hours. In rabbits and guinea-pigs such exposures can cause death (review by Lehmann & Flury, 1943).

As with other anaesthetics, prolonged anaesthesia with chloroform may result in respiratory depression, cardiac arrhythmia and finally in cardiac arrest. Heart failure is probably due to increased sensitivity of the heart muscle to adrenaline (Von Oettingen et al., 1950; Von Oettingen, 1964). Exposure of rabbits to 224 mg/m³ for 1 min led to decreased diastolic pressure, reduction of the stroke volume, blood pressure and cardiac output, and an increase in the peripheral vascular resistance. The cardiac effects were probably not due to respiratory effects, as blood oxygen and carbon dioxide tension and pH were not significantly changed (Taylor et al., 1976).

Exposure of rats to a chloroform concentration of 49 g/m³ for 5 h resulted in respiratory acidosis. Liver cells showed swollen rough endoplasmic reticulum with a loss of ribosomes, mitochondrial lesions, and cistern-like dilatation of tubular areas of the smooth endoplasmic reticulum. An accumulation of fat droplets and reduced amino acid incorporation into protein were also found in liver cells (Scholler, 1966, 1967).

Brondeau et al. (1983) found increased serum activities of glutamate dehydrogenase and sorbitol dehydrogenase after a single 4 h exposure of male rats to a chloroform concentration of 1410 mg/m³. The effects were dose-related and at the highest concentrations tested (4600 and 5250 mg/m³) serum aspartate aminotransferase levels (ASAT) were also increased.

7.1.2.4 Dermal exposure

Single application of 1 or 4 g chloroform/kg body weight for 24 h to the belly of rabbits, under an impermeable plastic cuff, resulted in extensive necrosis and weight loss at both levels. The kidneys of all animals showed dose-related degenerative changes in the tubules. Livers were not grossly affected (see also section 7.4) (Torkelson et al., 1976).

7.2 Short-term exposure

7.2.1 Oral exposure

7.2.1.1 Mice

Condie et al. (1983) dosed male CD1 mice daily with 0, 37, 74 and 148 mg chloroform/kg body weight in corn oil for 14 days. Histological changes turned out to be the most sensitive indicators of liver and kidney toxicity. Dose-related effects were observed at dose levels from 37 mg/kg body weight upwards. Kidneys showed intra-tubular mineralization, epithelial hyperplasia and cytomegaly. Livers showed centrilobular cytoplasmic pallor, marked cell proliferation and focal inflammation. After 14 days the body weight in the highest dose group was reduced.

Female and male CD1 mice (7-12 animals of each sex per group) were administered daily 0, 50, 125 and 250 mg/kg body weight in water by gavage for 14 and 90 days (Munson et al., 1982). Many histological and biochemical parameters were examined. After 14 days, the most important effects were a dose-related decrease in the number of antibody-forming cells (as IgM response to sheep red blood cells) in both sexes ($\geq$ 50 mg/kg body weight) and an increase in the liver weight of males at doses $\geq$ 125 mg/kg body weight and of females at the highest dose level. The serum ASAT level was increased in males and females at the highest dose level and serum ALAT was increased in females at the highest dose level. After 90 days, a depression in the number of antibody-forming cells was found at the highest dose level in both sexes. In females at the highest dose level, a decrease in cell-mediated type hypersensitivity was observed. Liver weight was increased after 90 days of exposure to doses $\geq$ 50 mg chloroform per kg body weight in the females and at 250 mg chloroform/kg body weight in the males. After 90 days of exposure, the animals showed a tolerance against a challenging dose of 1000 mg chloroform/kg body weight. The kidneys and livers of all dosed animals showed histological changes. In the kidneys these changes included small intertubular collections of chronic inflammatory cells, whereas in the liver they included generalized hydropic degeneration of hepatocytes and occasional small focal collections of lymphocytes. In females, small amounts of extravasated bile were occasionally noted in the sinusoidal Kupffer cells.

Jorgenson & Rushbrook (1980) administered chloroform to female B6C3F$_1$ mice for 90 days in the drinking-water at concentrations of 0, 200, 400, 600, 900, 1800 and 2700 mg/litre (measured daily chloroform doses of 0, 34, 66, 92, 132, 263 and 400 mg/kg body weight, respectively). In the first week of the experiment some mice in the higher dose groups died of dehydration due to reduced drinking. Depression of the central nervous system occurred in the animals receiving chloroform and was concentration-related. The only treatment-related histopathological findings consisted of a mild adaptive and transitory fatty change in the livers of animals dosed with 66 mg chloroform/kg body weight or more and a mild lymphoid atrophy of the spleen at the higher dose levels.

There is evidence that the vehicle in which chloroform is administered significantly affects its toxicity. Bull et al. (1986) found that chloroform administered by gavage in corn oil was significantly more hepatotoxic than equivalent doses administered in an aqueous emulsion (2% Emulphor®, polyoxyethylated vegetable oil, GAF Corp.). Doses of 0, 130 and 270 mg/kg were administered to male and female B6C3F$_1$ mice for 90 days. Liver body weight ratios were significantly higher in all dose groups and in both sexes when chloroform was administered in corn oil. The SGPT level was significantly elevated in both sexes at the high dose level of chloroform administered in corn oil, but not in those treated with the same dose in Emulphor. Mice treated at all levels of chloroform in corn oil showed evidence of extensive vacuolation and those treated with the high dose in corn oil showed extensive disruption of hepatic architecture including cirrhosis. No such pathological changes were observed in any of the animals treated with chloroform in 2% Emulphor.

One study contrasted the toxic responses of chloroform administered by gavage in corn oil or given *ad libitum* in the drinking-water (Larson et al., 1994a). Female B6C3F$_1$ mice were administered oral doses (0, 3, 10, 34, 90, 238, or 477 mg/kg per day) of chloroform dissolved in corn oil for 4 days or for 5 days/week for 3 weeks, or were continually exposed to chloroform in the drinking-water at concentrations of 0, 60, 200, 400, 900 or 1800 mg/litre for 4 days or 3 weeks, at which time they were necropsied. BrdU was delivered via osmotic pumps implanted 3.5 days prior to necropsy. Cell proliferation was evaluated as a BrdU labelling index (LI) in histological tissue sections. Dose-dependent changes included centrilobular necrosis and markedly elevated LI in mice given chloroform in corn oil at 238 or 477 mg/kg, the average daily doses that produced tumours in the gavage cancer bioassay (NCI, 1976a,b). The no-observed-effect level (NOEL) for histopathological changes was 10 mg/kg body weight per day and for induced cell proliferation 34 mg/kg body weight per day. Chloroform given in the drinking-water did not increase the hepatic LI after either 4 days or 3 weeks in any of the dose groups, nor were any microscopic alterations observed in the liver, even though the cumulative daily amount of chloroform ingested in the 1800-mg/litre exposure group was 329 mg/kg body weight per day (Larson et al., 1994a). Thus, the authors concluded that liver detoxification mechanisms are overwhelmed when chloroform is given as a single bolus dose, but the liver can detoxify the same daily dose if it is given in small amounts resulting from sips of water throughout the day. The authors also concluded that the sustained increase in LI in the livers of mice administered hepatocarcinogenic doses of chloroform in corn oil, but not in the case of chloroform in drinking-water, supports the hypothesis that chloroform-induced mouse liver cancer is secondary to events associated with induced cytolethality and cell proliferation (see also NCI, 1976a,b and section 7.7).

7.2.1.2 *Rats*

Chu et al. (1982a) exposed male weanling Sprague-Dawley rats to chloroform via drinking-water for 28 days. The following chloroform exposure doses were calculated: 0, 0.13, 1.3 and 11 mg/rat per day (0, 0.7, 7.4 and 63 mg/kg body weight, respectively). The only treatment-related effect observed was a decrease in the neutrophils in the 11-mg group. In a 90-day study by Chu et al. (1982b) male and female Sprague-Dawley rats were exposed to chloroform via drinking-water at dose levels of 0, 0.17, 1.3, 12 and 40 mg/rat per day for males and 0, 0.12, 1.3, 9.5 and 29 mg/rat per day for females; this was followed by 90 days of recovery. Water and food intake were reduced in the highest dose group. At the 40-mg level a higher incidence of spontaneous death occurred. Histological examination showed mild liver and thyroid lesions, especially in the highest dose group. Livers of both males and females showed: an increase in cytoplasmic homogeneity; density of the hepatocytes in the periportal area; mid-zonal and centrilobular increase in cytoplasmic volume; vacuolation due to fatty infiltration and occasional nucleic vesiculation; and hyperplasia of biliary epithelial cells. Thyroid lesions consisted of a reduction in follicular size and colloid density, increase in epithelial cell height and occasional collapse of follicles. Liver and thyroid lesions diminished in severity during the 90 days recovery period.

Jorgenson & Rushbrook (1980) administered chloroform in the drinking-water to male Osborne-Mendel rats for 90 days at concentrations of 0, 200, 400, 600, 900 and 1800 mg/litre (calculated to be 0, 20, 38, 57, 81 and 160 mg chloroform/kg body weight, respectively). A concentration-related central nervous system depression was seen. Body weights in the 160-mg group were reduced throughout the study. Biochemical investigations of serum showed no important deviations from control values other than a dose-related increase in cholesterol at dose levels of 38 mg chloroform/kg body weight or more after 60 days and a decrease in triglycerides in the highest dose group from 30 days onwards. After 90 days of administration, however, these parameters were affected in the two highest dose groups only. No dose-related histopathological changes were reported.

7.2.2 Inhalation exposure

The severity of liver injury due to inhaled chloroform is not only influenced by the administered concentration but also by the shape of the exposure profile. This was observed by Plummer et al. (1990), who exposed male black-hooded Wistar rats (36 per group) for 4 weeks to chloroform vapour as a constant concentration (245 mg/m^3; 24 h/day; 7 days a week) or as repeated concentrations (1387 mg/m^3; 6 h/day; 5 days a week), with a similar total exposure (154 g/m^3-hours) for the two ways of exposure (levels were monitored). Hepatic injury appeared to be more severe in the continuously exposed group, in which microvesicular fatty change was the most prominent feature, while focal necrosis was a minor feature. Livers of the animals receiving repeated exposures showed only minor injuries in the form of scattered hepatocytes containing small fat droplets and a few foci of liver cell necrosis.

Torkelson et al. (1976) exposed male and female rats (10-12 of each sex per group), rabbits (2-3 of each sex per group) and guinea-pigs (8-12 of each sex per group) to concentrations of 0, 110, 230 and 410 mg chloroform/m^3 air for 7 h/day, 5 days/week, during 6 months. In the male and female rats, relative kidney weight was increased at all exposure levels. In the males, at all levels, kidneys showed cloudy swelling of the tubular epithelium and the livers showed lobular granular degeneration with focal necrosis. At the higher exposure levels the effects became more pronounced. The effects observed in the males exposed to 110 mg chloroform/m^3 disappeared within 6 weeks after exposure. At 410 mg chloroform/m^3, death, due to interstitial pneumonitis, occurred in the males. No effects were seen in the male rats after 1, 2 or 4 h of exposure to 110 mg chloroform/m^3 (same schedule of exposure). The results obtained after exposure of rabbits and guinea-pigs were inconsistent because of low numbers of animals and/or the absence of dose-effect relationships.

The toxicity of one-week exposures to inhaled chloroform has been investigated in female B6C3F$_1$ mice and in male F-344 rats (Larson et al., 1994b; Méry et al., 1994). Rodents were exposed to chloroform vapour at concentrations of 0, 4.9, 14.7, 49, 147, 490 or 1470 mg/m³ (0, 1, 3, 10, 30, 100 or 300 ppm) for 7 consecutive days and necropsied on day 8. Cell proliferation was quantified as the percentage of cells in S-phase (BrdU labelling index) measured by immunohistochemical detection of BrdU-labelled nuclei. Mice exposed to 490 or 1470 mg/m³ exhibited centrilobular hepatocyte necrosis and severe vacuolar degeneration of mid-zonal and periportal hepatocytes, while exposure to 49 or 147 mg/m³ resulted in mild to moderate vacuolar changes in centrilobular hepatocytes. Slight, dose-related increases in the hepatocyte LI were observed for exposure concentrations of 4.9-14.7 mg/m³, while the LI was increased more than 30-fold in the 490- and 1470-mg/m³ groups. The kidneys of mice were affected only at 1470 mg/m³ exposure, with approximately half of the proximal tubules lined by regenerating epithelium and an 8-fold increase in the LI of tubule cells compared with controls (Larson et al., 1994b).

In rats, mild centrilobular vacuolation was observed only in the livers of animals exposed to 1470 mg/m³. The hepatocyte LI in rats was increased only at 490 and 1470 mg/m³ (3-fold and 7-fold over control, respectively). The kidneys of the male rats were affected only at 1470 mg/m³. About 25 to 50% of the proximal tubules were lined by regenerating epithelium in this exposure group, while the LI for tubule cells was increased 2-fold over controls (Larson et al., 1994b).

In the nasal passages of rats, chloroform concentrations of 49 mg/m³ or more induced histopathological changes that exhibited clear concentration-related severity. Chloroform-induced changes included increased epithelial mucosubstances in the respiratory epithelium of the nasopharyngeal meatus, primarily in the rats. A complex set of responses was seen in specific regions of the ethmoid turbinates, predominantly in the rats. These lesions in the ethmoid region, which involved all of the endo- and ectoturbinates, were most severe peripherally and generally spared the tissue adjacent to the medial airways. These changes were characterized by atrophy of Bowman's glands, increased numbers of vimentin-positive cells in the periosteum, new bone formation and increased number of periosteal cells in S-phase as determined by BrdU incorporation. Additional changes were site-specific loss of mucosubstances and loss of immunocyto-chemical staining of acini and ducts of Bowman's glands for P450-2E1 and pancytokeratin, and loss of P450-2E1 immuno-staining of the olfactory epithelium. The only change noted in the mice was increased periosteal cell proliferation without new bone growth (Méry et al., 1994).

7.3 Long-term exposure

In a carcinogenicity bioassay, female B6C3F$_1$ mice were exposed to 0, 200, 400, 900 or 1800 mg chloroform/litre drinking-water (number of animals: 430, 430, 150, 50 and 50, respectively) for a period of two years (Jorgenson et al., 1982) (see also section 7.7.1). These concentrations (monitored by analysis) correspond to time-weighted average daily chloroform doses of 0, 34, 65, 130 and 263 mg/kg body weight (Jorgenson et al., 1985). Matched controls (50 females) received an amount of water without chloroform equal to that consumed by the 1800-mg/litre group. Additional mice were used for intermediate biochemical and histopathological examination. Early mortality in the high-dose group was observed. After 3 months, livers of animals exposed to chloroform concentrations of 65 mg/kg body weight or more showed a higher fat content than those of the controls (as examined by chemical techniques). After 6 months, liver fat content was increased in all exposed groups. Data on organ weights were not provided.

In a carcinogenicity bioassay, male Osborne-Mendel rats were exposed to 0, 200, 400, 900 or 1800 mg chloroform/litre drinking-water (number of animals: 330, 330, 150, 50 and 50, respectively) for a period of two years (Jorgenson et al., 1982) (see section 7.7.2). These concentrations (monitored by analysis) correspond to time-weighted average daily chloroform doses of 0, 19, 38, 81 and 160 mg/kg body weight (Jorgenson et al., 1985). Matched controls received an amount of water without chloroform equal to that consumed by the 1800-mg/litre group. Additional rats were used for intermediate biochemical and histopathological examination. The survival was indirectly proportional to the dose levels. Concentration-related decreases in water uptake and growth were seen. The latter effects were also observed in the matched controls, and thus may be attributed to the reduced intake of water. Biochemical examination of blood after 6, 12 and 18 months showed that chlorine, potassium, total iron and albumin levels and the albumin/globulin ratio tended to be increased after chloroform treatment, whereas levels of cholesterol, triglycerides and lactate dehydrogenase were decreased in all treated groups. These deviations were also observed in the matched controls, but the decreases in serum triglycerides and cholesterol levels were more severe at the two highest dose levels than in the matched control group. Data on organ weights were not provided.

Beagle dogs were given chloroform in a toothpaste base in gelatin capsules, 6 days/week for 7.5 years (Heywood et al., 1979). The doses were 15 and 30 mg/kg and there were eight male and eight female dogs in each dose group. Dogs given the high dose began to show significant increases in SGPT levels at 6 weeks of treatment. At the low dose level, significant increases were observed at 34 weeks and after. Similar effects were not observed in the vehicle control (16 dogs of each sex) or untreated control (eight dogs of each sex) groups. "Fatty cysts" of the liver were observed in both dose groups at the end of this study (see section 7.7.3).

7.4 Skin and eye irritation

Adequate data on the skin irritation potential of chloroform has not been identified. Torkelson et al. (1976) applied liquid chloroform to the rabbit ear and found slight hyperaemia and exfoliation after one to four treatments (period between application and observation not specified). More frequent application did not increase the severity of the injuries. A 24-h application of chloroform on a cotton pad on the belly of rabbits produced slight hyperaemia, moderate necrosis and eschar formation. Chloroform delayed healing of mechanically damaged skin on the application site.

Application of chloroform droplets in the rabbit eye caused a transient slight irritation of the conjunctiva and corneal injury. A purulent exudate occurred for 2 or more days after the treatment (Torkelson et al., 1976).

Duprat et al. (1976) applied undiluted chloroform into the eyes of six New Zealand white rabbits. It produced severe eye irritation, with mydriasis and keratitis in all rabbits. Translucent zones in the cornea were observed in four animals and a purulent haemorrhagic discharge was also reported (number of rabbits unknown). The effects had disappeared 2-3 weeks after application, except for one rabbit that still showed corneal opacity after 3 weeks.

7.5 Reproductive toxicity, embryotoxicity and teratogenicity

7.5.1 Reproduction

Borzelleca & Carchman (1982) studied the reproductive toxicity of chloroform in a three-generation experiment with ICR mice.

They administered the chemical (0.1% Emulphor in deionised water) via drinking-water (in closed bottles) to males (10/group) and females (30/group), at concentrations of 0, 0.1, 1 and 5 mg/ml, from 5 weeks before F_0 mating throughout the entire study until sacrifice of the F_{2b} pups. Death occurred among the males and females of the highest dose group, and body weights in this group were reduced. At 1 mg/ml, the body weights of F_{1b} females were also reduced. Dose-related hepatotoxicity was found in the F_0 and F_{1b} animals (symptoms varying from "slight yellow-grey colouring" in the lowest dose group to "grey to black discolouration" with large nodules ($\geq$ 3 mm) upon and within the liver in the highest dose group). The treatment resulted in reduced fertility, litter size, gestation index and viability index in all F_1 and F_2 generations, statistically significant at 5 mg/ml. No evidence for a teratogenic potential was obtained.

7.5.2 Embryotoxicity and teratogenicity

Chloroform has not been found to be teratogenic but has been shown to induce fetotoxic effects.

7.5.2.1 Oral exposure

No evidence for a teratogenic effect of chloroform was obtained in a three-generation study with ICR mice (Borzelleca & Carchman, 1982).

In a study by Thompson et al. (1974), female Sprague-Dawley rats (25/group) were intubated with chloroform in corn oil (0, 10, 25 and 63 mg/kg body weight) twice daily on days 6-15 of gestation. A reduced body weight gain and anorexia were seen in the dams of the two higher dose groups. Tissues from two dams of each dose group were microscopically examined and fatty changes were observed in the livers of both females at 63 mg/kg and in one female at 25 mg/kg. Other signs of maternal toxicity were not found at these dose levels. The fetuses of the 63-mg/kg groups had a smaller weight at delivery than those of the control group. The incidence of bilateral extralumbar ribs was significantly increased among the fetal population of the 63-mg/kg dose group. Other minor visceral and skeletal abnormalities were seen, but not at significantly elevated levels. In the same study female Dutch-Belted rabbits (15/group) were dosed orally with chloroform in corn oil (0, 20, 35 and 50 mg/kg body weight) once daily during days 6-18 of gestation. Administration of chloroform produced a decrease in fetal body weight and incomplete ossification of skeletal elements (skull bones) in the 20- and 50-mg/kg dose groups. At the highest dose level the dams showed decreased weight gain. Signs of embryotoxicity and teratogenicity were not observed.

Ruddick et al. (1983) gave pregnant Sprague-Dawley rats (15/group) chloroform in corn oil (0, 100, 200 and 400 mg chloroform/kg body weight) daily by gavage from days 6 to 15 of gestation. All doses caused reduced weight gain in the dams and increased liver weight. At the highest dose level, there was an increase in the kidney weight of the dams. Haematological examinations showed dose-dependent reductions in haemoglobin and haematocrit (14% maximally, both parameters). In the highest dose group, the red blood cell count was also reduced.

According to Burkhalter & Balster (1979), oral administration of chloroform to mice from 3 weeks before mating until the end of the lactating period (in both sexes the dose was 31 mg/kg body weight) did not result in retardation of the development of responses to a battery of neurobehavioural tests in the pups.

7.5.2.2 Inhalation exposure

Schwetz et al. (1974) reported effects on pregnancy and on the incidence of fetal malformations in Sprague-Dawley rats exposed to chloroform concentrations of 147, 490 and 1470 mg/m^3 (30, 100 and 300 ppm) for 7 h/day during days 6-15 of gestation (analysis 3 times daily showed concentrations of 147, 466 and 1426 mg/m^3; 30, 95 and 291 ppm, respectively). The two highest concentrations were toxic to the dams (anorexia and reduced weight gain, increases in relative and absolute liver weight). There was a dose-dependent decrease in the pregnancy percentage (100% in the control group versus 15% in the 1426-mg/m^3 group) and in the number of living fetuses per litter. An increase was observed in the percentage of post-implantation losses (resorptions) in the highest dose group, and a dose-dependent increase was seen in the percentage of litters with resorptions (from 57% in the control group to 100% at the highest concentration). At all exposure levels, fetuses showed growth retardation and minor skeletal aberrations (delayed ossification of skull and sternebrae). Exposure to 147 mg/m^3 caused minor embryo- and fetotoxicity, and concentrations of 466 and 1426 mg/m^3 in the inhaled air were embryo- and fetotoxic to the rat. At the higher levels, subcutaneous oedema and other unspecified fetal soft tissue anomalies were also observed.

Murray et al. (1979) exposed pregnant CF1 mice (35-40/group) to 0 and 490 mg/m³ (0 and 100 ppm) for 7 h each day throughout days 1-7, 6-15 or 8-15 of gestation. The ability of females to maintain pregnancy was significantly decreased after exposure to chloroform during days 1-7 or 6-15 of gestation (44 and 43% in the treated groups versus 74 and 91% in the respective control groups). The dosed animals consumed slightly less food than the control animals, resulting in reduced body weight gain. Absolute and relative liver weights were increased in the groups exposed during days 6-15 and 8-15. After exposure during days 6-15, ALAT levels were significantly increased in pregnant and non-pregnant animals, the pregnant animals showing the smaller increase. Among the controls, no difference in ALAT activity was observed. An increase in total litter resorptions was observed after exposure through days 8-15. Mean fetal body weight and crown-rump length were decreased significantly if the dams had been exposed through days 1-7 or 6-15 of pregnancy. In the exposed groups an increased number of fetuses with delayed ossification of skull bones and sternebrae was observed, especially in the days 1-7 and 8-15 exposed groups. The incidence of cleft palates significantly increased in fetuses from dams exposed to 490 mg/m³ through days 8-15 of gestation for 7 h each day.

Published information for embryotoxicity and teratogenicity of chloroform in rat, mouse and rabbit by oral and inhalation exposure are summarized in Table 11.

7.6 Mutagenicity and related end-points

Very many genotoxicity assays have been conducted with chloroform and the data currently available are summarized in Tables 12 and 13. Some of these reports are from a large collaborative study comparing intra-laboratory variations in testing methodology (De Serres & Ashby, 1981).

Two problems potentially compromise the interpretation of mutagenicity data on chloroform. First, there is a possibility that ethyl and diethylcarbonate, produced by reaction of phosgene with ethanol that is routinely added to U.S.P (US Pharmacopoeia) chloroform, could generate false positive results. Secondly, testing of chloroform must be done in a sealed system because of its volatility, and so studies that did not take this factor into account could give false negative results.

Table 11. Embryotoxicity, fetotoxicity and teratogenicity produced in animals by exposure to chloroform

Species	Dose	Gestational days administered	Route of administration	Result	Reference
Rat	30, 100, 300 ppm	6-15 (7 h/day)	inhalation	embryotoxic fetotoxic	Schwetz et al. (1974)
Rat	20, 50, 126 mg/kg per day	6-15	oral	fetotoxic	Thompson et al. (1974)
Rat	100, 200, 400 mg/kg per day	6-15	oral	fetotoxic	Ruddick et al. (1983)
Mouse	100 ppm	1-7, 6-15, 8-15 (7 h/day)	inhalation	embryotoxic fetotoxic	Murray et al. (1979)
Rabbit	20, 35, 50 mg/kg per day	6-18	oral	fetotoxic	Thompson et al. (1974)

Table 12. Mutagenicity studies with chloroform

Species	Strain/cells	Measured end-point	Test conditions	Activation[a]	Inducer[b]	Result[c]	Reference
Bacterial systems							
Salmonella typhimurium	TA1535 TA1538	base-pair substitution frame-shift mutation	¹⁴C-labelled compound tested; no further details reported	+ ra	i.m., i.n.r.	-	Uehleke et al. (1976, 1977)
S. typhimurium	TA1535 TA1538	base-pair substitution frame-shift mutation	5 mM tested; incubation in closed containers (survival > 80%)	+ m	PB	-	Uehleke et al. (1976, 1977)
S. typhimurium	TA98 TA1537 TA1538 TA100 TA1535	frame-shift mutation frame-shift mutation frame-shift mutation base-pair substitution base-pair substitution	suspension test and vapour test; concentration in suspension test was 10% v/v, no further details	- + r	i.n.r.	- -	Simmon et al. (1977)
S. typhimurium	TA98 TA1537 TA1538 TA100 TA1535	frame-shift mutation frame-shift mutation frame-shift mutation base-pair substitution base-pair substitution	up to 3600 µg/plate; incubation in air-tight desiccators	- + r	PCB	- -	Gocke et al. (1981)

83

Table 12 (contd).

Species	Strain/cells	Measured end-point	Test conditions	Activation[a]	Inducer[b]	Result[c]	Reference
S. typhimurium	TA98 TA1537 TA1538 TA100 TA1535	frame-shift mutation frame-shift mutation frame-shift mutation base-pair substitution base-pair substitution	test conditions not reported	- + r	PCB	- -	Trueman (1981)
S. typhimurium	TA98 TA100	frame-shift mutation base-pair substitution	test conditions not reported	- +		- -	Ichinotsubo et al. (1981b)
S. typhimurium	TA98 TA100	frame-shift mutation base-pair substitution	0.5, 1.0, 5.0, 100, 200, 500 µg/plate	- + r	PCB	- -	Venitt & Crofton-Sleigh (1981)
S. typhimurium	TA98 TA1537 TA1535	frame-shift mutation frame-shift mutation base-pair substitution	microtitre fluctuation test; 1, 5, 10 µg/ml	- + r	PCB	- -	Gatehouse (1981)
S. typhimurium	TA98 TA100	frame-shift mutation base-pair substitution	fluctuation test; 1-500 µg/ml (not specified)	- + r		± -	Hubbard et al. (1981)
S. typhimurium	TA98 TA1537 TA1538 TA100 TA1535	frame-shift mutation frame-shift mutation frame-shift mutation base-pair substitution base-pair substitution	solvent DMSO; no further details	- + r	PCB	- -	Baker & Bonin (1981)

Table 12 (contd).

				- / + r		± / -	
S. typhimurium	TA98 TA1537 TA100 TA1535	frame-shift mutation frame-shift mutation base-pair substitution base-pair substitution	test conditions not reported	- + r	PB	± -	Garner et al. (1981)
S. typhimurium	TA98 TA1537 TA100	frame-shift mutation frame-shift mutation base-pair substitution	50, 100, 200, 1000, 2000, 5000 µg/plate	- + r	PCB	- -	MacDonald (1981)
S. typhimurium	TA98 TA1537 TA100	frame-shift mutation frame-shift mutation base-pair substitution	solvents DMSO; no further details	- + r	PCB	- -	Nagao & Takahashi (1981)
S. typhimurium	TA98 TA1537 TA1538 TA100 TA1535	frame-shift mutation frame-shift mutation frame-shift mutation base-pair substitution base-pair substitution	0.1, 1.0, 10, 100, 500, 2000 µg/plate; solvent DMSO	- + r	PCB	- -	Rowland & Severn (1981)
S. typhimurium	TA1535 TA1537 TA1538	base-pair substitution frame-shift mutation frame-shift mutation	10, 100, 1000, 10 000 µg/plate; solvent DMSO	- + r	PCB	- -	Richold & Jones (1981)
S. typhimurium	TA98 TA1537 TA1538 TA100 TA1535	frame-shift mutation frame-shift mutation frame-shift mutation base-pair substitution base-pair substitution	test conditions not reported	- + r	PCB	- -	Simmon & Shepherd (1981)

Table 12 (contd).

Species	Strain/cells	Measured end-point	Test conditions	Activation[a]	Inducer[b]	Result[c]	Reference
S. typhimurium	TA98 TA1537 TA1538 TA100 TA1535 TA92	frame-shift mutation frame-shift mutation frame-shift mutation base-pair substitution base-pair substitution interstrand DNA crosslinks	solvent DMSO or water; 0.2, 2, 20, 200, 2000 µg/plate	- + r	PCB	- -	Brooks & Dean (1981)
S. typhimurium	TA98 TA1537 TA1538 TA100	frame-shift mutation frame-shift mutation frame-shift mutation base-pair substitution	10, 100, 1000, 10 000 µg/plate	- + r + m	PCB PCB	- - -	Van Abbé et al. (1982)
S. typhimurium	TA1535 TA1538	base-pair substitution frame-shift mutation	vapour test; exposure for 2, 4, 6 or 8 h	- + r	PCB	- -	Van Abbé et al. (1982)
S. typhimurium	TM 677	forward mutation to azaguanine resistance	solvent DMSO; up to 300 µg/ml	+ r	PCB	-	Skopek et al. (1981)
Escherichia coli	WP2 uvrA	reversion to trp+	10, 100, 1000 µg/plate	+ r	PCB	-	Gatehouse (1981)
E. coli	WP2 uvrA	reversion to trp+	test conditions not reported	+ r	PCB	-	Matsushima et al. (1981)

Table 12 (contd).

Organism	Strain	Endpoint	Conditions	Result	Activation	Result	Reference
E. coli	WP2p WP2 uvrA	reversion to trp[+]	solvent acetone; 0.1, 1, 10, 100, 1000, 10 000 µg/plate	+ r -	PCB	- -	Kirkland et al. (1981)
E. coli	WP2p WP2 uvr p	reversion to trp[+]	0.5, 1.0, 5, 10, 50, 100, 200, 500 µg/plate	- + r	PCB	- -	Venitt & Crofton-Sleigh (1981)
E. coli	K12	base-pair substitution (not specified)	^{14}C-labelled compound tested; no further details reported	+ ra	i.m.	-	Greim et al. (1977)
Photobacterium phosphoreum	PPL⁻	reversion to normal light emission	disc-diffusion assay; no further details reported	-		+	Wecher & Scher (1982)

Non-mammalian eukaryotic systems

Organism	Strain	Endpoint	Conditions	Result	Activation	Result	Reference
Allium cepa		chromosomal aberrations	solvent: DMSO; 0, 250, 500, 1000, 1500, 2500, 5000, 10 000 µg/ml			+	Cortés et al. (1985)
Saccharomyces cerevisiae	D7	mitotic gene conversion at trp 5 locus	no details reported	+ n.r.	i.n.r.	-	Zimmermann & Scheel (1981)
S. cerevisiae	D7	mitotic gene conversion at trp 5; mitotic recombination at ade 2, reversion at ilv 1 loci	21, 41, 54 mM; incubation in screw-capped glass tubes	-		+	Callen et al. (1980)

Table 12 (contd).

Species	Strain/cells	Measured end-point	Test conditions	Activation[a]	Inducer[b]	Result[c]	Reference
S. cerevisiae	D6	mitotic aneuploidy	agar added	+ r	PCB	-	Parry & Sharp (1981)
S. cerevisiae	D6	mitotic aneuploidy	direct incubation in plastic bottles, 25, 50, 100 μg/ml; idem in glass bottles	+ r + r	PCB PCB	± -	Parry & Sharp (1981)
S. cerevisiae	JD1	mitotic gene conversion at trp 5 locus and his 5 polaron	up to 1000 μg/ml; incubation in plastic containers	+ r	PCB	±	Sharp & Parry (1981a)
S. cerevisiae	JD1	idem as above	idem as above, only incubation in glass containers	+ r	PCB	-	Sharp & Parry (1981a)
S. cerevisiae	D4	mitotic gene conversion at ade 2 and trp 5 loci	0.33, 1.0, 3.33, 100, 333.3 μg/plate	- + r	 PCB	- -	Jagannath et al. (1981)
S. cerevisiae	T1 T2	mitotic crossing over at ade 2	100, 1000 μg/plate	- + r	 PCB	- -	Kassinova et al. (1981)
S. cerevisiae	XV 185-14 C (haploid)	reversion at his 1, hom 3, and arg 4 loci	solvent DMSO; 111, 1111 μg/ml	- + n.r.	i.n.r.	- -	Mehta & Von Borstel (1981)

Table 12 (contd).

					PCB		
Schizosaccharomyces pombe	P1	forward mutation at ade 1, 3, 4, 5 and 9 loci	5, 7.5, 10 µg/ml	- + r		- (+)	Loprieno (1981)
Aspergillus nidulans	35 (haploid)	forward mutation (induction of methionine suppressors)	0.5% (survival 26%)	?		-	Gualandi (1984)
A. nidulans	P1	somatic segregation (crossing-over and non-disjunction)	0.5% (survival 16.5%)	?		-	Gualandi (1984)
Drosophila melanogaster	Berlin K wild and Basc	sex-linked recessive lethal test	Basc-test; 24 mM; adult feeding			-	Gocke et al. (1981)
D. melanogaster	Berlin K wild and y mei 9a mei-41 D5	sex-linked recessive lethal test	Basc-test; solvent DMSO; 0.1, 0.2% treated at 25 °C for 3 days with standard feeding technique			-	Vogel et al. (1981)
In vitro mammalian systems							
Chinese hamster	V79	forward mutation to 8-azaguanine resistance	1, 1.5, 2, 2.5%	-		-	Sturrock (1977)

89

Table 12 (contd).

Species	Strain/cells	Measured end-point	Test conditions	Activation[a]	Inducer[b]	Result[c]	Reference
Human	lympho-cytes	chromosome breakage	solvent acetone; 50, 100, 200, 400 µg/ml	+ r	PCB	-	Kirkland et al. (1981)
In vivo mammalian systems							
Mouse	CD1	micronuclei in polychro-matic erythrocytes of bone marrow	intraperitoneal, 0.015, 0.03, 0.06 ml/kg body weight at 0 and 24 h			-	Tsuchimoto & Matter (1981)
Mouse	NMRI	micronuclei in polychro-matic erythrocytes of bone marrow	intraperitoneal, 238, 476, 952 mg/kg body weight at 0 and 24 h			-	Gocke et al. (1981)
Mouse	B6C3F₁	micronuclei in polychro-matic erythrocytes of bone marrow	intraperitoneal, about 0.088 ml/kg body weight at 0 and 24 h or at 0 h only			-	Salamone et al. (1981)
Mouse	?	micronuclei in polychro-matic erythrocytes of bone marrow	route not reported; 100, 200, 400, 600, 700, 800, 900 mg/kg body weight			(+)	Agustin & Lim-Sylianco (1978)

Table 12 (contd)

Rat	Long-Evans	chromosomal aberrations in bone marrow	intraperitoneal, 1.2-119.4 mg/kg body weight; oral, 6-597 mg/kg body weight	+	Fujie et al. (1990)

Host-mediated assays

S. typhimurium	TA1535	base-pair substitution	test conditions not reported	-	Agustin & Lim-Sylianco (1978)
S. typhimurium	TA1537	frame-shift mutation	test conditions not reported	+	Agustin & Lim-Sylianco (1978)

[a] + = with metabolic activation
   - = without metabolic activation
   m = mouse
   r = rat
   ra = rabbit
   n.r. = species not reported
   ? = not reported if metabolic action was used

[b] PB = phenobarbital
   PCB = polychlorinated biphenyls
   i.m. = intact microsomes added
   i.n.r. = inducer not reported

[c] + = positive
   (+) = weakly positive
   ± = equivocal; study cannot be evaluated
   - = negative

Table 13. Indicator studies with chloroform

Species	Strain/cells	Measured end-point	Test conditions	Activation[a]	Inducer[b]	Result[c]	Reference
Bacterial systems							
Escherichia coli	WP2, WP67 uvrA pol A & CM 871 uvrA lexA recA	DNA damage (growth inhibition)	test concentrations not specified; no further details	- + r	PCB	- -	Tweats (1981)
E. coli	WP2, WP67 uvrA pol A & CM 871 uvrA lexA recA	DNA damage	test conditions not reported	-		-	Green (1981)
E. coli	W3110 (polA⁺), P3478 (POLA1)	DNA damage	liquid suspension test; 25 mg/ml; solvent DMSO or water	- + r	PCB	- (+)	Rosenkranz et al. (1981)

Table 13 (contd).

Organism	Strain	Endpoint	Test conditions	Result	Result	Result	Reference
E. coli	JC 2921 rec JC 9238 rec JC 8471 rec JC 5519 rec JC 7689 rec JC 7623 rec	DNA damage	test conditions not reported	+	−	+	Ichinotsubo et al. (1981a)
E. coli	56-161 env A C 600	induction of prophage λ in lysogenic *E. coli*	0.5, 5 mg/ml	+ r	PCB	− −	Thomson (1981)
Bacillus subtilis	H17 rec$^+$ M45 rec$^-$	DNA damage not further specified	maximum concentration: 20 µl/plate	+ r + yf + jc		− − −	Kada (1981)

Non-mammalian eukaryotic systems

Organism	Strain	Endpoint	Test conditions	Result	Result	Result	Reference
Allium cepa		SCE	solvent DMSO; 0, 250, 500, 1000, 1500, 2500, 5000, 10 000 µg/ml			±	Cortés et al. (1985)
Saccharomyces cerevisiae	T4 T5	DNA repair	solvent DMSO; 0.1, 1.0%	−			Kassinova et al. (1981)

Table 13 (contd).

Species	Strain/cells	Measured end-point	Test conditions	Activation[a]	Inducer[b]	Result[c]	Reference
S. cerevisiae	197/2d rad 3, rad 18, rad 52, trp 2	DNA repair	100, 300, 600, 750 µg/ml; incubation in plastic bottles	- +		± ±	Sharp & Parry (1981b)
In vitro mammalian systems							
Chinese hamster	ovary	SCE	0.7% (after exposure, 78% of dose remained)	+ r	PCB	-	White et al. (1979)
Chinese hamster	ovary	SCE	0.01, 0.1 µg/ml; solvent DMSO	+ r	PCB	-	Perry & Thomson (1981)
Chinese hamster	ovary	SCE	0.001, 0.01, 0.1 mM	-		+ [d]	Athanasiou & Kyrtopoulos (1981)
Rat	erythroblast	SCE	only 1.0 mM tested	+		(+)	Fujie et al. (1993)

Table 13 (contd).

Species	Tissue	Assay	Concentration			Reference
Syrian hamster	embryo	adenovirus transformation	0.12, 0.25, 0.50, 1.0, 2.0 ml/sealed chamber (4.6 litre)	-	+	Hatch et al. (1983)
Baby hamster	kidney	cell transformation	test conditions not reported	- + r	(+) -	Daniel & Dehnel (1981)
Baby hamster	kidney	cell transformation	0.25, 2.5, 25, 250 µl/ml	-	-	Styles (1979, 1981)
Rat	primary hepatocytes	UDS	0.00084-8.4 mM	-	-	Althaus et al. (1982)
Mouse (B6C3F$_1$)	primary hepatocyte	UDS	0.01-10 mM	-	-	Larson et al. (1994c)
Human	primary hepatocyte	UDS	4 cases 0.01-1.0 mM	-	-	Butterworth et al. (1989)
Human	lympho-cytes	SCE	0.016-50 mM	-	+	Morimoto & Koizumi (1983)

Table 13 (contd).

Species	Strain/cells	Measured end-point	Test conditions	Activation[a]	Inducer[b]	Result[c]	Reference
Human	lympho-cytes	SCE	solvent acetone; 25, 50, 75, 100, 200, 400 µg/ml	+ r	PCB	-	Kirkland et al. (1981)
Human	lympho-cytes	UDS	0.1, 1.0, 10 mM	- + r	PB	- -	Perocco et al. (1983)
Human	lympho-cytes	UDS	2.5, 5, 10 µg/ml	- + r	PB	- -	Perocco & Prodi (1981)
Human	Hela cells	UDS	0.1-100 µg/ml; solvent DMSO	- + r	PB	- -	Martin & McDermid (1981)
In vivo mammalian systems							
Mouse	JCR/SJ	SCE in bone marrow cells	oral: 25, 50, 100, 250 mg/kg body weight per day for 5 days			+	Morimoto & Koizumi (1983)
Mouse	B6C3F$_1$	DNA repair in liver	oral: 240 mg/kg body weight			-	Reitz et al. (1982)

Table 13 (contd).

Mouse	C57BL x C3H	sperm abnormalities	vapour exposure: 0.04, 0.08%; 4 h/day for 5 days	+	Land et al. (1981)
Mouse	CBA x BALB/C	sperm abnormalities	intraperitoneal: 0.025, 0.05, 0.075, 0.1, 0.25 mg/kg body weight per day for 5 days; vehicle corn oil	-	Topham (1980, 1981)
Rat	F-344	UDS in hepatocytes	oral: 40, 400 mg/kg body weight, single dose, vehicle corn oil	-	Mirsalis et al. (1982)
Mouse	B6C3F$_1$	UDS in hepatocytes	238, 477 mg/kg body weight, single dose, corn oil vehicle	-	Larson et al. (1994c)
Rat (neonatal)	liver and kidney cells	DNA damage (^{3}H elution)	vehicle corn oil; 200-400 mg/kg body weight	-	Petzold & Swenberg (1978)

[a] + = with metabolic activation; - = without metabolic activation; r = rat; yf = Yellowtail fish; jc = Japanese clam

[b] PB = phenobarbital; PCB = polychlorinated biphenyls

[c] + = positive; (+) = weakly positive; ± = equivocal; study cannot be evaluated; - = negative;

[d] In this test chromosome aberrations were also reported to occur; no details on this finding were reported.

In data presented in Table 12, three separate studies using the Ames assay were conducted under sealed conditions to assure chloroform retention. All three studies yielded negative test results.

In not all studies was it reported whether an *in vitro* assay was performed in a sealed chamber to prevent chloroform evaporation (Table 12). However, dimethylsulfoxide (DMSO) was often used as a solvent, thus increasing retention in the media. Furthermore, even in the case of an unsealed chamber, chloroform would be expected to stay in the media for a period of hours, and very high doses (up to 10 mg/plate) were often used.

Chloroform has been tested by a number of authors in validated bacterial systems with *Salmonella typhimurium* and *Escherichia coli* and showed to be negative both with and without metabolic activation. Only in one uncommon test with *Photobacterium phosphorum* was a positive effect found (Wecher & Scher, 1982).

The majority of studies with non-mammalian eukaryotic systems (yeasts and other fungi) were negative. Positive results were obtained with *Saccharomyces cerevisiae* D7, but only at the highest concentration tested, at which there was a marked toxic effect (Callen et al., 1980). It should be noted that this strain of yeast contains an endogenous cytochrome P450-dependent monooxygenase system. In *Schizosaccharomyces pombe* an indication for a mutagenic effect was observed (Loprieno, 1981). The inconsistent results with *Saccharomyces cerevisiae* D6 and JD 1 were probably due to inadequate test conditions (exposure in plastic rather than glass containers) and therefore it can be considered that chloroform was non-mutagenic in these tests (Parry & Sharp, 1981; Sharp & Parry, 1981a). In two sex-linked recessive lethal tests with *Drosophila melanogaster*, no mutagenic activity was observed (Gocke et al., 1981; Vogel et al., 1981).

Chloroform did not induce gene mutations in V79 Chinese hamster cells (Sturrock, 1977), or chromosomal aberrations in human lymphocytes *in vitro* (Kirkland et al., 1981).

In vivo mammalian testing comprised four micronucleus tests in mice, three of which gave a negative result (Tsuchimoto & Matter, 1981; Gocke et al.,1981; Salamone et al., 1981). The fourth micronucleus test was reported to have given a weakly positive result (Agustin & Lim-Sylianco, 1978). The same authors found a positive effect in the mouse host-mediated assay with *Salmonella typhimurium* TA1537 but not with TA1535.

Indicator studies showed that chloroform induces sister-chromatid exchange (SCE) in hamster and human cells *in vitro* in the absence of metabolic activation, and in mice *in vivo* (Athanasiou & Kyrtopoulos, 1981; Morimoto & Koizumi, 1983). Positive or weakly positive results were reported in two tests on DNA damage and DNA repair with *Escherichia coli* and *Saccharomyces cerevisiae* (Sharp & Parry, 1981b; Rosenkranz et al., 1981; Ichinotsubo et al., 1981a).

The ability of chloroform to induce unscheduled DNA synthesis (UDS) was examined in the *in vitro* and *in vivo* hepatocyte DNA repair assays for the most sensitive site for tumour formation, the female mouse liver (NCI, 1976a,b). In the *in vitro* assay, primary hepatocyte cultures from female B6C3F$_1$ mice were incubated with concentrations from 0.01 to 10 mM chloroform in the presence of ^{3}H-thymidine. UDS was assessed by quantitative autoradiography. No induction of DNA repair was observed at any concentration. In the *in vivo* assay, animals were treated by gavage with chloroform in corn oil (238 and 477 mg/kg body weight). Primary hepatocyte cultures were prepared 2 and 12 h later, incubated with ^{3}H-thymidine and assessed for induction of UDS. No DNA repair activity was seen at either dose or at either time point. These negative results in the target organ are consistent with the suggestion that neither chloroform nor its metabolites react directly with DNA *in vivo*.

The ability of chloroform to induce DNA repair was examined in freshly prepared primary cultures of human hepatocytes from discarded surgical material. No activity was seen in cultures from four different individuals at concentrations as high as 1 mM chloroform (Butterworth et al., 1989).

Given the large number of sensitive assays to which chloroform has been submitted, it is noteworthy that the reported positive responses are so few. Furthermore, these few positive responses were randomly distributed amongst the various assays with no apparent pattern or clustering for any test system. Taken together, the weight of evidence indicates that neither chloroform not its metabolites would appear to interact directly with DNA or possess genotoxic activity. The conclusion is consistent with the lack of initiating activity of chloroform (see section 7.7.4).

7.7 Carcinogenicity

7.7.1 *Mice*

In a National Cancer Institute carcinogenicity study, B6C3F$_1$ mice received USP grade chloroform stabilized with ethanol (0.5-1%) in corn oil 5 times a week by gavage (NCI, 1976a,b). Dosing was stopped after 78 weeks and the animals were sacrificed after 92 weeks. There were 20 animals per sex in the control group and 50 animals per sex in the dosed groups. The dose levels changed after 18 weeks, resulting in time-weighted average dose levels of 138 (low) and 277 (high) mg chloroform/kg body weight for male mice and 238 (low dose) and 477 (high dose) mg chloroform/kg body weight for female mice. Administration of the highest dose of chloroform reduced survival in the female mice. Causes of death were related to the observed liver tumours, pulmonary inflammation and cardiac thrombosis. This latter lesion was not observed in either the control or the low-dose group. Dose-related increased frequencies of hepatocellular carcinomas were found, the incidences being 1/18, 18/50 and 44/45 at 0, 138 and 277 mg chloroform/kg body weight in the males and 0/20, 36/45 and 39/41 at 0, 238 and 477 mg chloroform per kg body weight in the females, respectively. Mice presented clinical signs of illness, i.e. a reduced food intake and an untidy appearance, but clear information on non-neoplastic lesions was not provided. There is evidence that tumour formation may have been secondary to induced cytolethality and regenerative cell proliferation (see Larson et al., 1994a, and section 7.2.1.1).

Jorgenson et al. (1985) exposed female B6C3F$_1$ mice to chloroform in their drinking-water for a period of two years. The concentratións were 0, 200, 400, 900 and 1800 mg/litre, and the numbers of animals were 430, 430, 150, 50 and 50 per group, respectively. Time-weighted average daily doses were 0, 34, 65, 130 and 263 mg/kg body weight. Additional matched controls (50 animals) received the same quantity of drinking-water (without chloroform) as was consumed by the animals in the highest dose groups. Initially, 25% of the animals in the two highest dose groups died, but later on the death rate was more or less equal to that in the control group. No treatment-related effects on either liver or total tumour incidence were observed. Lack of tumour formation is consistent with the lack of induced liver necrosis or regenerative hepatocyte cell proliferation when chloroform is administered in the drinking-water (see Larson et al., 1994a and section 7.2.1.1).

The difference between the results obtained in the NCI study (1976a,b) and the Jorgenson et al. (1985) study is probably related to the manner in which the compound was administered. When given in the drinking-water, only small amounts of chloroform reach the liver, corresponding to each sip taken. Apparently, these small doses and delivery rates can be metabolized, detoxified and eliminated without liver damage (Larson et al., 1994a). When similar daily amounts are given as a single bolus dose in corn oil, it is probable that the high rate of delivery to the liver results in the production of toxic metabolites that overwhelm detoxification mechanisms, resulting in cell death and regenerative cell proliferation (Larson et al., 1994a). The choice of vehicle may also contribute to the observed difference in toxicity (Bull et al., 1986) (see also section 7.2.1.1).

Roe et al. (1979) administered daily chloroform (British Pharmacopoeia quality) in a toothpaste base (vehicle) to ICI mice (control group 104 animals per sex, dose groups 52 animals per sex) by gavage, 6 days a week for 80 weeks, followed by a 16-week observation period. The dose levels were 0 (controls), 17 and 60 mg/kg body weight. Mice that died during the first 15 weeks of the experiment were replaced by animals from a reserve group (which were probably also dosed, although this was not specified). The control toothpaste did not contain eucalyptol and peppermint oil, whereas the toothpaste containing chloroform did contain these substances. Treatment with chloroform resulted in slightly increased survival, especially in the males. The most common cause of death was respiratory failure. A slightly increased incidence of fatty degeneration was observed among the chloroform-treated animals. Total tumour incidence was increased in the male mice (20/37 and 21/38 at 17 and 60 mg/kg body weight, respectively, versus 20/72 in the controls). Renal tumours (3 hypernephromas and 5 cortical adenomas) were reported in 8 out of 38 males of the high-dose group.

In a second experiment by Roe et al. (1979), the influence of peppermint oil, eucalyptol and chloroform was determined separately. In this study, male ICI mice received 60 mg chloroform/kg body weight daily, in the same way as in the study reported above. The vehicle control (toothpaste without chloroform, eucalyptol and peppermint oil) and dose groups consisted of 260 and 52 male animals, respectively (the groups receiving a dose of peppermint or eucalyptol also consisted of 52 animals). Again, the survival in the chloroform-dosed group was better than in the control group. Total tumour incidence was lower in the chloroform-treated group (30/49 versus 170/240 in the controls). However, administration of chloroform resulted in a kidney tumour frequency (hypernephromas and adenomas) of 9/49, compared with a control value of 6/240.

In a third study by Roe et al. (1979), 60 mg chloroform/kg body weight in toothpaste (containing eucalyptol and peppermint oil) was administered daily to male mice (52 per group) of the ICI, CBA, C57BL and the CF1 strain for a period of 80 weeks. The chemical was also administered in arachis oil to male mice of the ICI strain. Each strain had its own control group. Terminal sacrifice was at 93, 97-99, 104 and 104 weeks for the CF1, ICI, C57BL and CBA strains, respectively. In this study, a treatment-related increase in the survival was found in all strains tested, except for the CF1 strain. Treatment with chloroform resulted in a higher incidence of renal changes in the CBA and CF1 strains but not in the C57BL strain. The cause of death in all four strains was renal neoplasia in combination with respiratory and renal disease. In the C57BL, CBA and CF1 strains no changes in tumour frequencies were observed. In the ICI mice, after treatment with chloroform in either the toothpaste vehicle or arachis oil, an increase in the incidence of malignant kidney tumours was found (3/47 versus 0/49 in the controls, toothpaste vehicle; 9/48 versus 0/50 in the controls, arachis oil vehicle).

Though full results are not yet available, an additional carcinogenesis bioassay in which mice were exposed to chloroform by inhalation is under way (Matsushima, personal communication, 1993).

7.7.2 Rats

In a National Cancer Institute carcinogenicity study, Osborne-Mendel rats received USP grade chloroform stabilized with ethanol (0.5-1%) in corn oil 5 times a week by gavage (NCI, 1976a,b). Dosing was stopped after 78 weeks and the animals were sacrificed after 111 weeks. There were 20 animals per sex in the control group and 50 animals per sex in the dosed groups. The dose levels changed after 23 weeks, resulting in time-weighted average dose levels of 90 (low dose) and 180 (high dose) mg chloroform/kg body weight for males and 100 (low) and 200 (high) mg chloroform/kg body weight for females. Administration of chloroform reduced survival in male and female rats in all dose groups. A clear pathological reason for this effect in the rats was not given. In male rats, dose-related increased frequencies of kidney epithelial tumours were observed (incidences: 0/19, 4/50 and 12/50 at 0, 90 and 180 mg chloroform/kg body weight, respectively). In the females a non-significant increase in the frequency of thyroid tumours was found (incidences: 1/19, 8/49 and 10/46 at 0, 100 and 200 mg chloroform/kg body weight, respectively). Rats presented clinical signs of illness, i.e. a reduced food intake and an untidy appearance. However, clear information on non-neoplastic lesions was not provided.

Reuber (1979) re-evaluated the histological sections of the NCI study (1976a,b) and reported the same neoplastic lesions as the NCI. In addition, he noted that chloroform-dosed female rats developed liver lesions that were not seen in the control females (i.e. cholangiofibromas 0/20, 1/39 and 3/39; cholangiocarcinomas 0/20, 2/39 and 8/39; hyperplastic nodules 1/20, 7/39 and 12/39; and hepatocellular carcinomas 0/20, 2/39 and 2/39, for the control, low- and high-dose groups, respectively).

Jorgenson et al. (1985) exposed male Osborne-Mendel rats via drinking-water to 0, 200, 400, 900 and 1800 mg chloroform/litre for a period of two years. Time-weighted average daily chloroform doses were 0, 19, 38, 81 and 160 mg/kg body weight and the numbers of animals were 330, 330, 150, 50 and 50 per group, respectively. Additional matched controls (50 animals) received the same quantity of drinking-water (without chloroform) as was consumed by the animals in the highest dose groups. As a probable consequence of reduced drinking and reduced body weights, death rate was reduced with increasing chloroform dosage and in the matched control group. The only dose-related effect was an increase in renal tubular cell adenomas and adenocarcinomas. The incidence for all kidney tumours was 5/301, 1/50, 6/313, 7/148, 3/48 and 7/50 for control, matched control and the 19, 38, 81 and 160 mg/kg groups, respectively. From 38 mg/kg body weight upwards the increase in the frequency of all kidney tumours was statistically significant.

In an inadequately reported study, Tumasonis et al. (1985) exposed male and female Wistar rats to 0 or 2900 mg chloroform per litre drinking-water during the lifetime of the animals. Animal numbers were 26 and 22 in the male and female control groups and 32 and 45 in the male and female treated groups, respectively. The experiment started with weanlings. After 72 weeks, the drinking-water chloroform concentrations were reduced because of an increased intake of water by exposed animals. However, daily intakes of chloroform varied considerably and so the time-weighted average daily doses were estimated roughly from a figure in the report. They appeared to be around 180 mg/kg body weight in the males and around 240 mg/kg body weight in the females. Body weights were decreased and life-span was increased in the exposed animals. A severe hepatic adenofibrosis (cholangiofibrosis) was observed in the exposed animals. Ten out of the 40 females examined showed hepatic hyperplastic nodules (none did in the control group). In the males no increase in the incidence of neoplastic nodules was found.

Although full results are not yet available, an additional carcinogenesis bioassay in which rats were exposed to chloroform by inhalation is under way (Matsushima, personal communication, 1993).

7.7.3 Dogs

Heywood et al. (1979) administered chloroform to Beagle dogs at dose levels of 0, 15 and 30 mg/kg body weight (6 days/week) in toothpaste in a gelatin capsule for a period of 7.5 years. Sacrifice followed after an observation period of 19 to 23 weeks, during which the chloroform treatment was withdrawn. The control group consisted of 16 animals of each sex and the dose groups of 8 animals of each sex. There were no treatment-related increases in tumours.

7.7.4 Studies on initiating-promoting activity

7.7.4.1 Mice

One week after a single intraperitoneal administration of ethylnitrosourea (0, 5 or 20 mg/kg body weight) to 15 days old CD1 Swiss mice (both sexes), Pereira et al. (1985) exposed the animals to chloroform via drinking-water at concentrations of 0 or 1800 mg/litre until they were 51 weeks of age, after which the animals were sacrificed. The chloroform treatment did not affect the liver or lung tumour frequency in the females and the lung tumour frequency in the males. However, the liver tumour frequency in the males appeared to be reduced after the treatment.

Capel et al. (1979) administered chloroform as a drinking-water solution (estimated daily doses of 0, 0.15 or 15 mg/kg body weight) to male mice either from 14 days before or from 14 days before to 14 days after intraperitoneal injection with Ehrlich ascites cells (TO strain), subcutaneous injection with B16 melanoma cells (C57BL strain) or intramuscular injection with Lewis lung carcinoma cells (C57BL strain). Chloroform treatment enhanced the growth of Ehrlich ascites cells (measured as intraperitoneal tumour cell DNA) at the high dose level. In comparison with the controls, more animals receiving chloroform at both dose levels had organs invaded with B16 melanoma cells. Lewis lung tumour growth, measured as primary tumour size or pulmonary metastases, was not significantly enhanced at low-dose chloroform treatment, but after treatment with the high dose the number of pulmonary metastases and tumour size were markedly increased.

In a two-stage (initiation/promotion) treatment protocol, Klaunig et al. (1986) studied the effect on liver tumour incidence in male B6C3F$_1$ mice (35/group) after continuous treatment with 600 and 1800 mg chloroform/litre drinking-water for 52 weeks to determine if chloroform expresses its hepatocarcinogenicity through tumour promotion mechanisms. Two groups received 600 and 1800 mg chloroform/litre drinking-water containing diethylnitrosamine (DENA; 10 mg/litre) during the first 4 weeks of exposure. Two other groups received 600 and 1800 mg chloroform/litre drinking-water without DENA. The DENA groups constituted the initiated groups. One initiated and one non-initiated control group were included. Chloroform did not affect the incidence of liver or lung tumours by itself, and even inhibited liver and lung tumorigenesis in the DENA-initiated mice, compared with DENA treatment alone.

7.7.4.2 *Rats*

Deml & Oesterle (1985, 1987) studied the ability of chloroform to promote the development of liver tumours. Female Sprague-Dawley rats were initiated for liver tumours by administration of a single dose of 8 mg dimethyl nitrosamine/kg body weight. This was followed by administering chloroform (25, 100, 200 and 400 mg/kg body weight) in an olive oil vehicle twice weekly for 11 consecutive weeks. There was a dose-related increase of ATPase-negative, γ-glutamyl transpeptidase (GGTase)-positive and glycogen-storing foci of cells within the liver. For example, ATPase-deficient foci were increased from approximately 2-fold to 5-fold by doses of 100 and 400 mg/kg, respectively. These data demonstrate that chloroform in an oil vehicle will probably promote development of hepatic tumours in rats.

Herren-Freund & Pereira (1986) evaluated the ability of chloroform to act as an initiator, promoter and co-carcinogen in B6C3F$_1$ mice and male Sprague-Dawley rats. In rats, the initiator was administered 18-24 h following a two-thirds partial hepatectomy. Diethylnitrosamine (0.5 mmol/kg body weight) was used as the positive control for initiation and phenobarbital (500 mg/litre drinking-water) was used as the positive control for promotion. Ethylnitrosourea (ENU) was the positive control for initiator in 15-day-old mice and phenobarbital (500 mg/litre drinking-water) was used as the positive control for promotion. Chloroform was administered as a single dose of 180 and 360 mg/kg body weight as an initiator (no vehicle) in the rat and 1800 mg/litre drinking-water for 48 weeks as a promoter. There was no evidence that chloroform was able to act as an initiator in rats. Moreover, it did not act as a tumour promoter in either mice or rats, but actually decreased the numbers of hepatic tumours induced in neonatal mice by ENU. Concurrent administration of chloroform and DENA to the rat had no significant effect on foci or tumour development in rats. These data further suggest that the corn oil vehicle is important to the hepatocarcinogenic effects of chloroform.

In a previous experiment, Pereira et al. (1982) had examined the effect of chloroform as an initiator and promoter. Chloroform was administered at 180 mg/kg body weight in a single dose as an initiator and 180 mg/kg body weight twice a week for 53 days as a promoter. In this case, tricaprylin was the vehicle. Chloroform had no activity as an initiator. There was a small, but statistically significant, increase in the numbers of GGTase-positive foci in the promotion study.

Although chloroform is an established rodent carcinogen, several studies have shown that chloroform administered in impolar solvents also has anti-cancer properties as it inhibits tumour growth in mouse liver and in the gastrointestinal tract of the rat (Pereira et al., 1985; Daniel et al., 1989).

Chloroform administered in drinking-water (0, 900 and 1800 mg/litre) to Fischer-344 rats significantly decreased gastrointestinal (GI) tumours that were initiated by a single 200 mg/kg dose of dimethyl hydrazine (DMH) (Daniel et al., 1989). GI tumour incidence was 14/39 in animals treated with DMH alone and 5/39 and 5/40 in the groups in which DMH treatment was followed by 900 and 1800 mg chloroform/litre, respectively, for 39 weeks.

Chloroform also inhibits the propensity for three gastrointestinal tract carcinogens, benzo(a)pyrene (BAP), 1,2-dimethylhydrazine (DMH) and methylnitrosourea (MNU), to induce nuclear anomalies in the proximal colon of B6C3F$_1$ mice (Daniel et al., 1991). These authors found that in mice pre-adapted to 1800 mg chloroform/litre drinking-water for 30 days prior to the carcinogen administration the level of nuclear anomalies induced in the proximal colon was reduced by four-fold for BAP and two-fold for both MNU and DMH. In the duodenum, chloroform was effective at inhibiting unclear anomalies only for MNU.

Reddy et al. (1992) demonstrated that chloroform inhibits the development of diethylnitrosamine-initiated, phenobarbital-promoted γ-glutamyl transpeptidase and placental form glutathione-S-transferase-positive foci in the liver of male Fischer-344 rats. They suggested that chloroform exerts its focal inhibitory effect by selectively killing the putative initiated cells.

The lack of initiating activity in these initiation-promotion assays supports the conclusion that chloroform is non-genotoxic (section 7.6), and also indicates that the carcinogenic action of chloroform is attributable to a non-genotoxic/cytotoxic mode of action (sections 7.2.1.1 and 7.7). Interestingly, more of the above studies reported that chloroform inhibited the growth or formation of precancerous or cancerous cells than those that reported that chloroform had promotional activity.

7.8 In vitro studies

In vitro studies frequently provide insight into how chemicals induce cytotoxic effects. However, at high concentrations (e.g., 5 mM and above), the solvent effects of chloroform on cell membranes complicate the interpretation of these experiments. The preparations that have been studied are precision-cut slices taken from the liver, primary hepatocytes suspensions and cultures.

Azri-Meehan et al. (1992) studied the cytotoxic effects of chloroform in liver slices taken from phenobarbital-treated rats. No comparison was made with non-induced animals. Concentrations in the range of 0.5 to 1.6 mM induced loss of intracellular potassium and glutathione. Reduced mitochondrial function (measured as decreases in dye reduction) was observed in the same dose range. A concentration of 0.2 mM had no effect.

Glende & Recknagel (1992) examined the ability of a number of chlorinated hydrocarbons to activate phospholipase A_2, presumably through damage to calcium-binding sites in the endoplasmic reticulum. At doses that induce 30 to 70% release of cellular lactate dehydrogenase (i.e. 9.8 mM), chloroform did activate phospholipase A_2. This concentration is similar to that necessary to destroy the calcium-binding capacity of the endoplasmic reticulum.

O'Hara et al. (1991) examined the effects of chloroform on the viability of hepatocytes in suspension (measured by potassium retention). These hepatocytes were isolated from control phenobarbital-treated rats. The minimum concentration required to produce an effect on potassium retention decreased from 10 mM in control hepatocytes to 1 mM in hepatocytes obtained from induced animals.

A number of studies of chloroform cytotoxicity in suspensions of rat hepatocytes have been reported (Stacey, 1987). However, the very high nominal concentrations of chloroform that were apparently necessary to produce significant effects (i.e. 30 and 60 mM) raise considerable questions as to their relevance to *in vivo* hepatic toxicity.

An innovative approach has been developed for incubating hepatocyte suspensions with the chemical of interest, followed by observation of the cytotoxic response after placing the treated cells into culture (Kedderis et al., 1993a). Such cytotoxicity was observed when hepatocyte suspensions derived from B6C3F$_1$ mice were incubated with concentrations of chloroform between 1.3 and 3.8 mM. These concentrations were consistent with peak liver concentrations expected with the high doses of chloroform utilized in the assessment of chloroform carcinogenicity in mice (NCI, 1976a,b), as predicted by the Corley et al. (1990) pharmacokinetic model (Kedderis et al., 1993b). The cytotoxicity of chloroform was potentiated by pretreating the mice with acetone to induce cytochrome P450 2E1.

Although there have been substantial advances in the study of *in vitro* chloroform toxicity, the applicability of the results that are available to date to estimate hazards in humans remains to be established.

7.9 Factors modifying toxicity; toxicity of metabolites

The *in vivo* toxicity of chloroform is modified by a range of factors. The rate of its biotransformation is a significant determinant of its toxicity. Hence, factors that increase or decrease chloroform biotransformation may alter the intensity of chloroform-induced toxicity. The activities of the cytochrome P450 isoforms that catalyse the biotransformation of chloroform differ among species and between sexes of experimental animals. Moreover the activities of the enzymes that metabolize chloroform may be increased or decreased by exposure to chemicals, and exposure to chloroform itself may alter chloroform metabolism.

In addition to differences in the rates of chloroform bioactivation, treatments that alter susceptibility are also important determinants of chloroform-induced toxicity. Cellular glutathione concentrations are an important determinant of susceptibility, and perturbations of glutathione homeostasis may affect markedly the toxicity of chloroform. Finally, for some of the treatments that alter chloroform toxicity discussed in this section, the mechanistic basis of these interactions is not well understood.

Brown et al. (1974a) reported that inhalation exposure of phenobarbital-treated male Sprague-Dawley rats to chloroform at doses of 2.45 or 4.9 g/m³ (500 or 1000 ppm) for 2 h produced marked centrilobular necrosis that was accompanied by decreased hepatic glutathione concentrations. *In vitro* studies showed that glutathione reduced the covalent binding of [^{14}C]-chloroform metabolites to microsomal protein.

Docks & Krishna (1976) observed that administration of chloroform decreased hepatic glutathione concentrations in phenobarbital-treated rats (male, Sprague-Dawley), but not in control animals 1 to 2 h after administration, and caused liver necrosis. Administration of isopropanol or acetone, which increased the covalent binding of chloroform metabolites (Sipes et al., 1973), did not alter hepatic glutathione concentrations.

Starvation and carbohydrate restriction increase the *in vivo* metabolism of chloroform and its hepato- and nephrotoxicity in rats (Nakajima & Sato, 1979; McMartin et al., 1981; Nakajima et al., 1982). In contrast, protein deficiency does not alter chloroform toxicity (McLean, 1970).

Several authors have demonstrated that administration of alcohols, including ethanol (Kutob & Plaa, 1962b; Sato et al., 1980, 1981), or ketones increases chloroform metabolism and hepatotoxicity. An extension of these studies to include a range of alcohols showed that methanol, ethanol, isopropanol, *tert*-butanol, pentanol, hexanol, octanol and decanol all potentiate chloroform-induced liver injury and lower the LD_{50} of chloroform in male Sprague-Dawley rats (Ray & Mehendale, 1990). Aliphatic ketones, including acetone, 2-butanone, 2-pentanone, 2-hexanone, 2,5-hexanedione, 2-heptanone and methyl isobutyl ketone, also increase chloroform-induced hepatotoxicity (Hewitt et al., 1990; Vézina et al., 1990), but treatment with 2-hexanone does not increase chloroform-dependent lipid peroxidation either *in vivo* or *in vitro* (Cowlen et al., 1984a,b). The potentiating effect of alcohols and ketones in chloroform-induced hepatotoxicity is attributed to an increase in the activity of the cytochromes P450 that metabolize chloroform (Koop et al., 1982; Ryan et al., 1986; Brady et al., 1989; Vézina et al., 1990).

Harris et al. (1982) evaluated, by the intraperitoneal route, the toxicity of chloroform (0.2 ml/kg body weight) and carbon tetrachloride (0.1 ml/kg body weight) given alone or together to male rats. At these doses, neither chloroform nor carbon tetrachloride produced toxicity, but increases in SGPT activity and hepatic triglyceride and calcium concentrations were seen when both compounds were given together. Ikatsu & Nakajima (1992) showed that a single inhalation exposure to 490 mg/m³ (100 ppm) chloroform for 8 h resulted in mid-zonal hepatotoxicity. In ethanol-treated rats exposed to both chloroform (50 ppm) and carbon tetrachloride (10 ppm), liver necrosis and elevated plasma GOT/GPT activities were observed. These findings indicate that the toxicity of chloroform is elevated in the presence of carbon tetrachloride. O'Hara et al. (1991) studied the effect of chloroform and carbon tetrachloride in rat hepatocytes and demonstrated that the combined toxicity of both compounds was greater than additive.

The pesticide kepone (chlordecone), but not its non-ketonic analogue mirex, increases chloroform-induced hepato- and nephrotoxicity (Hewitt et al., 1979, 1982; Iijima et al., 1983). In Mongolian gerbils, which are susceptible to chloroform-induced toxicity (200 or 500 μl/kg body weight, intraperitoneal), treatment with phenobarbital or chlordecone decreased the hepatotoxicity of chloroform (Ebel et al., 1987); in contrast, rats given 50 to 500 μl/kg body weight chloroform (intraperitoneally) showed little hepatotoxicity, but toxicity was increased after treatment with phenobarbital or chlordecone.

The drinking-water contaminants dichloroacetic acid (DCA) and trichloroacetic acid (TCA) potentiate chloroform toxicity (Davis, 1992). Male and female rats (Sprague-Dawley) were orally treated with 0.92 or 2.45 mmol/kg body weight DCA or TCA and were given 0.75 mg/kg body weight chloroform (intraperitoneally) 3 h later. Increases in plasma ALAT activities were observed in female, but not in male rats 24 and 48 h after giving DCA; in contrast, plasma ALAT activities were increased 24, but not 48 h, after giving TCA in both male and female rats. DCA administration increased blood urea nitrogen concentrations in female rats, but produced little effect in male rats, whereas TCA administration produced an effect only in female rats 48 h after treatment. The mechanism of the effect of DCA and TCA was not elaborated.

Monochloroacetic acid (MCA) given by gavage to male (188 mg/kg body weight) or female (94 mg/kg body weight) Sprague-Dawley rats one hour before giving chloroform (520 mg/kg body weight) intraperitoneally increased chloroform-induced hepatotoxicity in male rats, but had little effect in female rats (Davis & Berndt, 1992). Treatment with MCA alone decreased glomerular filtration rates in female rats. The mechanism by which MCA potentiated chloroform toxicity was not elucidated.

Temporal variations in chloroform-induced hepatotoxicity have been observed in rats (Lavigne et al., 1983). Male Sprague-Dawley rats were given chloroform (0.5 ml/kg body weight) intraperitoneally at 9:00, 13:00, 17:00, 21:00 or 03:00 h and were killed 4 h after treatment. Hepatotoxicity, as assessed by serum GPT, GOT and LDH activities, was minimal and maximal at 09:00 h and 21:00 h, respectively, whereas glucose-6-phosphatase activity was decreased at 03:00 h and 13:00 h. When rats were starved for 16 h before giving chloroform at 09:00 h, toxicity was increased substantially.

Charbonneau et al. (1991) studied the effect of acetone treatment on the toxicity with a range of binary mixtures of haloalkanes in rats. An increased hepatotoxic response was observed with binary mixtures containing chloroform, carbon tetrachloride, 1,1,2-trichloroethane or 1,1-dichloroethylene.

In vitamin-A-deficient rats, serum ALAT and particularly ASAT activities were increased after intraperitoneal administration of chloroform, compared to control rats (Savoure et al., 1992).

8. EFFECTS ON HUMANS

8.1 Acute non-lethal effects

Chloroform is irritating to mucous membranes, producing gastroenteritis with persistent nausea and vomiting. Symptoms following ingestion of chloroform are similar to those following inhalation (van der Heijden et al., 1986).

Cases of severe intoxication after suicidal attempts, with the same pattern of symptoms as after anaesthetical use, have been reported by Schröder (1965). There are considerable inter-individual differences in susceptibility. Some persons presented serious illness after an oral dose of 7.5 g of chloroform, whereas others survived a dose of 270 g chloroform. The mean lethal dose for an adult is estimated to be about 45 g (Winslow & Gerstner, 1978).

Rao et al. (1993) successfully managed acute toxicity from chloroform in a 33-year-old white woman who attempted suicide by injecting 0.5 ml of chloroform, and then drank half a cup the next morning. Plasma chloroform levels, measured by headspace GC, declined rapidly. Sequential measurement of biomarkers in serum for liver cell necrosis, liver function and liver regeneration indicated the presence of initial liver damage followed by recovery. The authors suggested that, in addition to biomarkers for liver necrosis, serial determinations of markers for liver regeneration provide objective evidence for recovery from chloroform poisoning.

It has been reported that chloroform can cause severe toxic effects in humans exposed to 9960 mg/m^3 (2000 ppm) for 60 min, symptoms of illness at 2490 mg/m^3 (500 ppm) and can cause discomfort at levels below 249 mg/m^3 (50 ppm) (Verschueren, 1983).

Most data on the controlled exposure of man to chloroform have resulted from its clinical use as an anaesthetic. This use of chloroform was described as early as 1847 (Simpson, 1847). Induction of anaesthesia may result from inhalation of chloroform vapours at a concentration of 24 to 73 g/m^3 air. For maintenance of anaesthesia, concentrations in the range of 12 to 48 g/m^3 are required. As with animals, chloroform anaesthesia may result in death in humans due to respiratory and cardiac arrhythmias and failure. Because of the relatively high frequency of "late chloroform poisoning" (liver toxicity), its use as anaesthetic has been abandoned.

Other effects related to chloroform inhalation are: increase in the rate and depth of respiration during induction and light anaesthesia, minute volume decrease in deep anaesthesia, hypothermia, depletion of adrenal adrenaline content, hypotension, depression of gastrointestinal tract motility, respiratory acidosis, hyperglycaemia, ketosis, constriction of the spleen, increase in the number of leucocytes (especially polymorphonuclear cells), a decrease in clotting time and an increase in prothrombin time. The characteristics and severity of the effects depend on depth and duration of anaesthesia (Adriani, 1970).

The cardiac effects might be secondary and due to hypoxia, caused by depression of respiratory activity. No studies have been found in which this problem has been investigated in man (e.g., by forced respiration), but Taylor et al. (1976) obtained indications that chloroform itself produces cardiovascular disturbances in rabbits (viz. disturbances in left ventricular functioning and an increase in peripheral resistance; see section 7.1.2.3) after exposure to 244 mg/m^3 for 1 min.

In man, as well as in animals, renal tubular necrosis and renal dysfunction (anuria, proteinuria, uraemia, increase in blood urea nitrogen) have been observed (Kluwe, 1981). Recovering from chloroform anaesthesia, some patients may show the symptoms of a delayed chloroform poisoning several days later. Prostration, protracted nausea, vomiting, jaundice and coma due to hepatic dysfunction are observed. The patient may die within 5 days after anaesthesia. At autopsy, degeneration and necrosis of liver tissue have been found (Goodman & Gilman, 1970). In general the symptoms appear to be similar to those observed in animals.

According to Oettel (1936) and Winslow & Gerstner (1978), exposure to concentrated chloroform vapours causes a stinging sensation in the eye. Splashing of the liquid into the eye evokes burning, pain and redness of the conjunctival tissue. Occasional injury of the corneal epithelium will recover fully within a few days. Dermal contact with chloroform causes chemical dermatitis (symptoms: irritation, reddening, blistering and burns).

8.2 Epidemiology

8.2.1 *Occupational exposure*

Challen et al. (1958) reported the effects of exposure of workers (mostly female) to chloroform vapour in a factory during manufacture of lozenges containing the chemical. Eight workers (four working full-time and four half-time) were exposed to chloroform concentrations of 375 to 1330 mg/m³, with a peak concentration of 5680 mg chloroform/m³, for periods of 3 to 10 years. The symptoms reported were lassitude, thirst, gastrointestinal distress, frequent and scalding urination, lack of concentration, depression and irritability. The management stated that some of the employees had been noticed staggering about at work. Nine other workers (one full-time, eight half-time), who were exposed to chloroform concentrations of 110 to 350 mg/m³ for 10 to 24 months, suffered from the same complaints as stated above, but to a lesser degree. Several liver function tests did not reveal signs of liver toxicity, but these tests were not very sensitive.

Bomski et al. (1967) investigated the occurrence of hepatitis in a chemical factory in relation to the occurrence of this disease in the city where the factory was located. The 68 workers were exposed to occupational chloroform concentrations of 10 to 1000 mg/m³ for 1 to 4 years. In this group of employees, a higher frequency of hepatitis was found than in the city inhabitants. Seventeen workers showed hepatomegaly and in three of them hepatitis was observed. Ten workers showed splenomegaly, but the cause of the splenomegaly was not discussed.

The finding of a high frequency of hepatitis among occupationally chloroform-exposed workers, as compared to that in the city inhabitants, is supported by a recent report on a 16-year-old patient who attempted suicide by ingesting chloroform. This led to the development of toxic hepatitis (Hakim et al., 1992).

In a study by Phoon et al. (1975), the air in the workroom of 13 persons with jaundice originally diagnosed as having viral hepatitis was analysed for chloroform. The chloroform concentration in the workroom appeared to be more than 1950 mg/m³. The period of exposure was less than 6 months. Because no worker had a history of fever and there was no relation to past medical history, it was concluded that the original diagnosis must have been wrong and should have been toxic jaundice. Five of the people with jaundice and four other colleagues had blood chloroform levels in the range of 1 to 2.9 mg/litre.

In another factory 18 cases of what seemed to be hepatitis B were reported (Phoon et al., 1983). Investigation of the occupational environment revealed a constant exposure to chloroform, with concentrations in the range of 80 to 160 mg/m³. The exposure period of these workers was less than 4 months and the conclusion was drawn that these were cases of toxic jaundice related to chloroform exposure, because no infection with the hepatitis B virus could be established.

A historical mortality study was carried out by Linde & Mesnick (1979). They investigated the cause of death of white male anaesthesiologists, who were occupationally exposed to chloroform vapours (extent of exposure was unknown). The death certificates used were of persons, who were presumed to be exposed during the 1880-1890 period and who died during the 1930-1946 period. Comparison of their death certificates with those of several control groups did not exclude a possible association between cancer and chloroform exposure.

8.2.2 General exposure

There have been numerous reports over the last 15 years which have evaluated the relationship between chlorinated water and the incidence of cancer. Chloroform is but one of many by-products produced by reaction of chlorine with naturally occurring material in source waters (Bull & Kapfler, 1991). Many of these studies noted increased risk of cancer which at least partially fulfilled criteria for causality (e.g., consistency, specificity and temporal relationships).

IARC (1991) reviewed the available studies and concluded the strongest evidence of increased risk related to exposure to chlorinated surface water relative to unchlorinated ground water for the incidence of cancer of the urinary bladder. However, the weight-of-the-evidence evaluation by IARC concluded that there is inadequate evidence for the carcinogenicity of chlorinated drinking-water in humans.

Morris et al. (1992) conducted a meta-analysis which attempted to integrate quantitatively the results of previously published studies in which individual exposures were evaluated (i.e. case control and cohort studies). The authors identified increased rates of bladder and colo-rectal cancer in individuals exposed to chlorinated surface water, which appeared to exhibit a dose-related trend. Although this study was confounded by substantial differences in exposure variables that occur in different water supplies, higher risk rates were estimated when the analysis was restricted to those studies which were judged to have the highest quality exposure assessments. Because of the confounding of these results by chlorine residual levels and a multiplicity of other chemicals which are animal carcinogens and mutagens, none of the drinking-water studies specifically implicate chloroform as a human carcinogen.

Kramer et al. (1992) studied the association between exposure to trihalomethanes in the water supply and adverse reproductive outcomes in the state of Iowa (USA). Estimations of chloroform exposure were based on municipal water surveys. After adjustment for maternal age, parity, prenatal care, marital status, education and maternal smoking, an increased risk for intra-uterine growth retardation (abnormally low birth weight) was associated with chloroform concentrations above 10 μg/litre. Limitations of the study involve the ascertainment and classification of exposures to trihalomethanes (such as fluctuation of levels and exposure at individual level) and the influence of potential confounding influences of unmeasured contaminants.

8.3 Abuse and addiction

Exposure to chloroform may result in euphoria and therefore people expose themselves to chloroform by drinking the liquid or sniffing the vapours (Storms, 1973). Addiction to chloroform and chloroform-containing cough syrups has been reported by Heilbrunn et al. (1945) and Conlon (1963). According to Heilbrunn et al. (1945), addicts tolerated very high daily doses and presented neurological symptoms and degenerative changes in the brains.

After an intravenous injection of 7.5 g of chloroform, a patient showed signs of pulmonary malfunction and haemolysis. In this case, kidney or liver toxicity was not reported (Timms et al., 1975).

9. EFFECTS ON OTHER ORGANISMS IN THE LABORATORY AND FIELD

9.1 Freshwater organisms

The data on the toxicity of chloroform to several freshwater organisms are listed in Table 14.

Due to the volatility of chloroform, caution must be exercised in interpreting the test results, particularly those in open static systems where no chemical analysis of the actual concentration was carried out.

9.1.1 Short-term toxicity

The chemical is of low toxicity to unicellular plants and other microorganisms (concentration range of initial population growth inhibition: 125 to > 3200 mg/litre). Chloroform is moderately toxic to *Daphnia magna* (LC_{50} = 29 mg/litre).

The LC_{50} values for several species of fish are in the range of 18 to 191 mg/litre. However, initial toxicity may occur at lower levels: the no-observed- lethal concentrations (NOLCs) for *Salmo gairdneri* and *Lepomis macrochirus* appear to be 8 and 3 mg/litre, respectively. At lower concentrations ($\leq$ 13 mg/litre), *Salmo gairdneri* shows loss of equilibrium, slow operculum movement and narcosis (Anderson & Lusty, 1980).

In *Gasterosteus aculeatus*, chloroform produced anaesthesia which could be maintained for at least 90 min at concentrations of 210 mg/litre. Exposure to concentrations higher than 300 mg/litre resulted in decreased oxygen consumption and death (Jones, 1947), whereas concentrations lower than 120 mg/litre excited the animals and gave rise to considerable higher oxygen uptake.

Chloroform is considerably more toxic to the juvenile stages of several species of amphibians. In a continuous-flow system, Birge et al. (1980) tested the toxicity of chloroform to embryo-larval stages of several species of amphibians after exposure for 7-9 days (Table 14). *Hyla crucifer* appeared to be the most susceptible species. An effect was found on the hatching rate of the embryos, which declined from 97% at 8 µg/litre to 4% at 7340 µg/litre. In addition there was some evidence of teratic larvae. During the 4 days post-hatching the LC_{50} declined from

Table 14. Chloroform toxicity to water organisms

Organism	Temperature (°C)	Medium	Stat/ flow[a]	Analysis[c]	Exposure duration	Parameter	Concentration (mg/litre)	Reference
Short-term toxicity								
Bacteria								
Pseudomonas putida	25	acc.[d] Bringmann & Kuhn (1977)	S	-	16 h	initial reduction of cell multiplication	125	Bringmann & Kühn (1977)
Pseudomonas fluorescens	25	acc.[d] Bringmann (1973)	S	-	16 h	intial change of culture turbidity	125	Bringmann (1973)
Algae								
Microcystis aeruginosa	27	acc.[d] Bringmann (1975)	S	-	192 h	initial reduction of cell multiplication	185	Bringmann (1975)
Scenedesmus quadricauda	25	acc.[d] Bringmann & Kuhn (1977)	S	-	192 h	initial reduction of cell multiplication	1100	Bringmann & Kühn (1977)
Haematococcus pluvialis	20	acc.[d] Tumpling (1972)	S	-	4 h	10% reduction of oxygen production	440	Knie et al. (1983)
Protozoans								
Entosiphon sulcatum	25	Bringmann (1978)	S	-	72 h	initial reduction of cell multiplication	> 6560	Bringmann (1978)

Table 14 (contd).

Organism	Temperature (°C)	Medium	Stat/flow[a]	Analysis[c]	Exposure duration	Parameter	Concentration (mg/litre)	Reference
Protozoans (contd).								
Uronema parduczi	25	Bringmann & Kühn (1980)	S	-	20 h	initial reduction of cell multiplication	> 6560	Bringmann & Kühn (1980)
Chilomonas paramaecium	20	Bringmann et al. (1980)	S	-	48 h	initial reduction of cell multiplication	> 3200	Bringmann et al. (1980)
Crustaceans								
Daphnia magna	22	reconstituted well water, pH 7, hardness 173 mg CaCO$_3$/litre	S	-	48 h	LC$_{50}$	29	LeBlanc (1980)
Daphnia magna	19.8–20.9	lake water, pH 8.0, hardness 157 mg CaCO$_3$/litre	S	-	48 h	LC$_{50}$	65.7	Gersich et al. (1986)
Daphnia magna	23	distilled water	S	-	48 h	LC$_{50}$	78.9	Abernethy et al. (1986)

Table 14 (contd)

Fish			S	A				
Cyprinus carpio (mixed gametes)	26	filtered well water	S	-	until hatching (3-5 days)	LC_{50}	97	Mattice et al. (1981)
Pimephales promelas (10-15 days)	25	carbon filtered lake water, pH 7.6-8.3, hardness 125 mg $CaCO_3$/litre	S	-	96 h	LC_{50}	129	Mayes et al. (1983)
(30-35 days)	22	idem	S	-	96 h	LC_{50}	171	
(60-100 days)	22	idem	S	-	96 h	LC_{50}	103	
Brachydanio rerio	20	dechlorinated tap water, pH 8, hardness 10 d.H.	CF	-	48 h	LC_{50}	100	Slooff (1979)
Salmo gairdneri	20	dechlorinated tap water, pH 8, hardness 10 d.H.	CF	-	48 h	initial reduction of respiration frequency	20	Slooff (1979)
Leuciscus idus melanotus	20	acc.[d] Mann (1975)	S	-	48 h	LC_{50}	162-191	Juhnke & Lüdemann (1978)
Carassius auratus	5	aerated tap water	S	-	1 h	EC_{50} (anaesthesia)	97-167	Cherkin & Catchpool (1964)
	20	aerated tap water	S	-	1 h	EC_{50} (anaesthesia)	167	

121

Table 14 (contd).

Organism	Temperature (°C)	Medium	Stat/flow[a]	Analysis[c]	Exposure duration	Parameter	Concentration (mg/litre)	Reference
Salmo gairdneri	19	aerated river water	CF	A	96 h	LC$_{50}$ NOLC	18 8	Anderson & Lusty (1980)
Leopomis macrochirus	19	aerated river water	CF	A	96 h	LC$_{50}$ NOLC	18 3	Anderson & Lusty (1980)
Micropterus salmoides	19	aerated river water	CF	A	96 h	LC$_{50}$ NOLC	51 39	Anderson & Lusty (1980)
Ictalurus punctatus	19	aerated river water	CF	A	96 h	LC$_{50}$ NOLC	75 68	Anderson & Lusty (1980)
Amphibians *Hyla crucifer* (eggs; 2 to 6 h post-spawning)	20.5	acc.[d] Birge et al. (1979); pH 7.6, hardness 107 mg CaCO$_3$/litre	CF	A	until 4 days after hatching or death (7 days in total)	LC$_{50}$	0.3	Birge et al. (1980)
	20.5	*idem*	CF	A	*idem*	NOLC	0.009	

122

Table 14 (contd).

Rana pipiens (eggs; 30 min after fertili- zation)	20.5	*idem*	CF	A	*idem* (9 days in total)	LC$_{50}$	4.2	Birge et al. (1980)
	20.5	*idem*	CF	A	*idem*	NOLC	0.16	
Rana palustris (eggs; 2 to 6 h post-spawning)	21.5	acc.[d] Birge et al. (1979); pH 7.6, hardness 104 mg CaCO$_3$/litre	CF	A	*idem* (8 days in total)	LC$_{50}$	20.6	Birge et al. (1980)
	21.5	*idem*	CF	A	*idem*	NOLC	0.33	
Bufo fowleri (eggs; 2 to 6 h post-spawning)	21.5	*idem*	CF	A	*idem* (7 days in total)	LC$_{50}$	35.1	Birge et al. (1980)
	21.5	*idem*	CF	A	*idem*	NOLC	0.33	
Long-term toxicity								
Fish *Poecilia reticulata*	22	Alabaster & Abram (1964)	S[b]	-	14 days	LC$_{50}$	102	Könemann (1981)

Table 14 (contd).

Organism	Temperature (°C)	Medium	Stat/flow[a]	Analysis[c]	Exposure duration	Parameter	Concentration (mg/litre)	Reference
Salmo gairdneri (eggs; 20 min after fertilization)	13.5 ± 1	acc.[d] Birge et al. (1979); pH 7.3, hardness 48 mg CaCO₃/litre	CF	A	until 4 days after hatching or death (27 days totally)	LC₅₀	2.0	Birge et al. (1979)
	13.5 ± 1	*idem*	CF	A	*idem*	NOLC	0.004	
	13.5 ± 1	*idem*, hardness 210 mg CaCO₃/litre	CF	A	*idem*	LC₅₀	1.24	
	13.5 ± 1	*idem*	CF	A	*idem*	NOLC	0.003	

[a] S = static, CF = continuous flow;
[b] static conditions but test water changed every 24 h
[c] A = concentration of test compound analysed during assay; - = no data
[d] acc. = according to the medium described in these references

124

760 to 270 μg/litre. The other species tested were less affected and only *Rana pipiens* showed a high teratogenicity frequency in the offspring (100% at 27 mg/litre at 18% hatching rate).

9.1.2 Long-term toxicity

Birge et al. (1979) tested the toxicity of chloroform for embryo-larval stages of *Salmo gairdneri* (Table 14) after 27 days. The chemical was especially toxic for the unhatched embryos (LC_{50} is about 2 mg/litre), but did not cause death in the larvae at concentrations up to 10.6 mg/litre. The occurrence of teratic survivors in the hatched population increased from 3% at 56 μg/litre to 40% at 10 mg/litre.

9.2 Marine organisms

The acute toxicity of chloroform to *Artemia salina* was tested by Robinson et al. (1965). The observed effect was anaesthesia and the EC_{50} value was 68 mg/litre after 10 h of exposure in artificial sea water in closed containers under static conditions. The 50% immobilization concentration (IC_{50}) of chloroform for *Artemia salina* nauplii, subjected to salinity stress, was determined in a static study using artificial sea water by Foster & Tullis (1985). The toxicity test began 30 h after hatching had commenced and lasted for 24 h. The IC_{50} was 37 mg/litre.

Stewart et al. (1979) tested the acute toxicity of chloroform to larvae of *Crassostrea virginica*. Chemical analysis showed a rapid decline of chloroform concentrations in the sea-water medium. The estimated LC_{50} was 1 mg/litre.

Pearson & McConnell (1975) tested the acute toxicity to *Limanda limanda* in a continuous-flow system containing natural sea water and obtained an LC_{50} of 28 mg/litre.

Cowgill et al. (1989) determined the sensitivity of the marine diatom *Skeletonema costatum* to chloroform after exposure for 5 days under static conditions. The EC_{50} values calculated were 477 mg/litre and 437 mg/litre based on total cell count and total cell volume, respectively. The NOEC was 216 mg/litre.

10. EVALUATION OF HUMAN HEALTH RISKS AND EFFECTS ON THE ENVIRONMENT

10.1 Evaluation of human health risks

10.1.1 Exposure

Based on estimates of mean exposure from various media, the general population is exposed to chloroform principally in food (approximately 1 µg/kg body weight per day), drinking-water (approximately 0.5 µg/kg body weight per day) and indoor air (0.3 to 1 µg/kg body weight per day). Estimated intake from outdoor air is considerably less (0.01 µg/kg body weight per day). The total estimated mean intake for the general population is approximately 2 µg/kg body weight per day. Available data also indicate that water use in homes contributes considerably to levels of chloroform in indoor air and to total exposure. For some individuals living in dwellings supplied with tap water containing relatively high concentrations of chloroform, estimated total intakes are up to 10 µg/kg body weight per day.

Workers may be exposed to chloroform during, for example, the production of chloroform itself, the synthesis of substances derived from chloroform (for example, chlorodifluoromethane), and the use of chloroform as a solvent, and also as a consequence of its formation in paper bleaching and sewage treatment facilities. For example, based on a national survey conducted from 1981 to 1983, NIOSH estimated that approximately 96 000 workers in the USA are potentially exposed to chloroform.

10.1.2 Health effects

The most important effects of chloroform are those on the liver and kidney. These effects are associated with the metabolism of chloroform to the reactive intermediate, phosgene. There are substantial interspecies and sex differences in the rates at which chloroform is metabolized. Data also indicate that reductive metabolism differs among species.

The most universally observed toxic effect of chloroform is damage to the liver. The severity of these effects per unit dose administered depends on the species, the vehicle and the method by which the chloroform is administered. The lowest dose at which liver damage has been observed is 15 mg/kg body weight per day, administered to beagle dogs in a toothpaste base over a period of 7.5 years. Effects at lower doses were not examined. Somewhat higher doses are required to produce hepatotoxic effects in other species. Although duration of exposure varied in these studies, no-observed-adverse-effect levels (NOAELs) ranged between 15 and 125 mg/kg body weight per day.

Effects on the kidney have been observed in male mice of sensitive strains and in F-344 rats. Severe effects have been observed in a particularly sensitive strain of male mice at doses as low as 36 mg/kg body weight per day.

Daily 6-h inhalation of chloroform for 7 days consecutively induced atrophy of Bowman's glands and new bone growth in the nasal turbinates of F-344 rats. The NOEL for these effects was 14.7 mg/m^3 (3 ppm). The significance of these effects is being further investigated in longer term studies.

The weight of the available evidence indicates that chloroform has little, if any, capability to induce gene mutation, chromosomal damage and DNA repair. There is some evidence of low-level binding to DNA, however. Chloroform does not appear capable of inducing unscheduled DNA synthesis *in vivo*.

Chloroform induced hepatic tumours in mice when administered by gavage in corn oil. However, when similar doses were administered in drinking-water to mice, hepatic tumours were not induced.

The carcinogenic effects of chloroform on the mouse liver appear to be closely related to cytotoxic and cell replicative effects. The effects on cell replication paralleled variations in carcinogenic responses to chloroform due to vehicle and method of administration. It is of interest, in this regard, that chloroform administered in drinking-water was incapable of promoting, but rather inhibited, the development of liver tumours in mice. Chloroform does not appear capable of initiating liver tumours or inducing unscheduled DNA synthesis in the mouse liver. It would appear, therefore, that cytotoxicity followed by cell replication with prolonged administration of chloroform is associated with the development of liver tumours in mice.

Chloroform induced kidney tumours in rats when administered by gavage in corn oil. However, results for this species were similar when the chemical was administered in the drinking-water.

Experiments in F-344 rats have indicated that chloroform could cause damage and increase cell replication in the kidney at doses similar to those that induce renal tumours in Osborne-Mendel rats. These effects are produced by both oral (one single gavage) and 7-day inhalation exposure. While these results are suggestive of an association, it is difficult to associate with any certainty the carcinogenic response with the toxic and replicative effects. Indeed, toxicity studies are short term and involve a rat strain that is unusually sensitive to the nephrotoxic effects of chloroform. This strain is different from that in which tumours were observed.

There are some limited data to suggest that chloroform is toxic to the fetus, but only at doses that are maternally toxic.

10.1.3 Approaches to risk assessment

The following guidance is provided as a potential basis for the derivation of exposure limits by relevant authorities. By allocation of the tolerable and risk-specific intakes presented below based, for example, on the proportion of total intakes originating from each environmental medium presented in chapter 5, limits for exposure in drinking-water, food and air could be developed by local authorities (WHO, in press). However, local authorities may also wish to take into account local variations in the proportions of exposure from various media or factors such as cost, ease and effectiveness of control in order to develop risk management strategies appropriate for local circumstances. However, the ultimate objective should be reduction of total exposure from all sources to levels below the tolerable maximum intake and risk-specific intakes presented below. Moderate to short-term excedence of limits based on the guidance presented below does not necessarily imply significant risk to health and relevant public health authorities should be contacted before taking remedial action.

Moreover, disinfection is unquestionably the most important step in the treatment of water for public supply. The paramount importance of microbiological quality requires some flexibility in the derivation of limits for exposure to chloroform in drinking-water. Where local circumstances require that a choice must be made between meeting microbiological limits or limits for disinfection byproducts, the microbiological quality must always take precedence. Efficient disinfection must *never* be compromised.

.1.3.1 Non-neoplastic effects

The Task Group concluded that the data available are sufficient to develop a tolerable intake for non-neoplastic effects of chloroform on the basis of effects in animal species.

The lowest effect level in long-term studies in animal species is that reported by Heywood et al. (1979) where slight hepatotoxicity (increases in hepatic serum enzymes and fatty cysts) was observed in beagle dogs that ingested 15 mg/kg body weight per day in toothpaste for 7.5 years. Liver fat content was also increased in B6C3F$_1$ mice that ingested 34 mg/kg body weight per day in drinking-water for 2 years (Jorgenson et al., 1985). On the basis of these data, a tolerable daily intake (TDI) can be derived as follows:

$$\text{TDI} = \frac{15 \text{ mg/kg body weight per day}}{1000} = \begin{array}{l} 0.015 \text{ mg/kg body weight per day} \\ (15 \text{ } \mu\text{g/kg body weight per day}) \end{array}$$

where:

- 15 mg/kg body weight per day is the lowest-identified-effect level (slight hepatotoxicity in the study on beagle dogs by Heywood et al., 1979);

- 1000 is the uncertainty factor (x 10 for interspecies variation, x 10 for intraspecies variation and x 10 for use of an effect level rather than a no-effect level).

This value is likely to be conservative. It should be noted that no effects have been observed in adequate studies on other species exposed to higher doses administered in other vehicles.

1.3.2 Neoplastic effects

The Task Group concluded that the carcinogenic effects of chloroform should also be considered in the development of limits of exposure.

a) Liver tumours in female B6C3F₁ mice

Based on the available mechanistic data, the approach considered most appropriate for provision of guidance based on mouse liver tumours is division of a no-effect level for cell proliferation by an uncertainty factor. The NOEL for cytolethality and cell proliferation in $B6C3F_1$ mice was 10 mg/kg body weight per day following administration in corn oil for 3 weeks (Larson et al., 1994a).

On the basis of these data, a tolerable daily intake is derived as follows:

$$TDI = \frac{10 \text{ mg/kg body weight per day}}{1000} = \begin{array}{l} 0.01 \text{ mg/kg body weight per day} \\ (10 \text{ } \mu\text{g/kg body weight per day}) \end{array}$$

where:

- 10 mg/kg body weight per day is the NOEL for cytolethality and cell proliferation in $B6C3F_1$ mice observed in the short-term study of Larson et al. (1994a);

- 1000 is the uncertainty factor (x10 for interspecies variation, x10 for intraspecies variation and x 10 for severity of effect (i.e. carcinogenicity) and less-than-chronic study).

b) Kidney tumours in male Osborne-Mendel rats

Since data on cell proliferation are not available for the strain in which tumours were observed (Osborne-Mendel rats) and identified information on cell proliferation and lethality are short term (one single gavage and a 7-day inhalation exposure in F-344 rats), it was considered premature to deviate from the default model (i.e. linearized multistage) as a basis for estimation of lifetime cancer risk.

Based on the induction of renal tumours (adenomas and adenocarcinomas) in male rats in the study by Jorgenson et al. (1985), the total daily intake considered to be associated with a 10^{-5} excess lifetime risk, calculated on the basis of the Global 82 version of the linearized multistage model, is 0.0082 mg/kg body weight per day (8.2 μg/kg body weight per day). A body surface area correction was not incorporated due to the fact that chloroform is an indirect-acting carcinogen and that the rate of metabolism is similar in rodents and man.

10.2 Evaluation of effects in the environment

Chloroform may be released into the environment during its production, storage, transport and use. Significant amounts of chloroform may also enter the environment as a consequence of its formation during some chlorination processes (e.g., chlorination of water, paper bleaching).

Chloroform is expected to volatilize readily from surface water and the surface of soils. It is also expected to be highly mobile in soils and may reach ground water.

Chloroform has a residence time of several months in the atmosphere and can therefore be transported over long distances from the point of emission. Degradation by reaction with hydroxyl radicals is likely to be the only significant mechanism for decomposition of chloroform in the atmosphere. A half-life of around 60 days has been estimated for this process.

Chloroform appears to be resistant to biodegradation under aerobic conditions but is degraded under certain anaerobic conditions.

Chloroform is toxic to the embryo-larval stages of some amphibian and fish species. The lowest reported LC_{50} is 0.3 mg/litre (4- or 7-day exposure) for the embryo-larval stages of *Hyla crucifer*. It is less toxic to fish and *Daphnia magna*. The LC_{50} values for several species of fish are in the range of 18 to 191 mg/litre. There is little difference in sensitivity between freshwater and marine fish. The lowest reported LC_{50} for *Daphnia magna* is 29 mg/litre (48-h exposure). Chloroform is of low toxicity to algae and other microorganisms.

Levels of chloroform in surface water are generally low and would not be expected to present a hazard to aquatic organisms. However, higher levels of chloroform in surface water resulting from industrial discharges or spills may be hazardous to the embryo-larval stages of some aquatic species.

11. FURTHER RESEARCH

A number of further studies is considered to be necessary:

- A study of compensatory cell regeneration in the liver and kidney of the Osborne-Mendel rat

- Determination of reactive metabolite formation *in situ*

- Studies on the mechanism of the species-specific carcinogenicity of chloroform including a) the identification of the intermediate/metabolite responsible for the carcinogenicity of chloroform and b) its mode of action

- An inhalation carcinogenicity bioassay

- Further validation of PBPK models for chloroform with interspecies variations, including humans and dogs

- Further studies concerning the progression of nasal lesions in the rat

- Additional long-term toxicity tests in aquatic organisms

- *In vitro* cytotoxicity/metabolism studies with human tissues

12. PREVIOUS EVALUATION BY INTERNATIONAL BODIES

The International Agency for Research on Cancer evaluated chloroform in 1978 (IARC, 1979) and re-evaluated it in 1987 (IARC, 1987). The conclusions were that there is inadequate evidence for the carcinogenicity of chloroform in humans but sufficient evidence for its carcinogenicity in experimental animals. The overall evaluation was that chloroform is possibly carcinogenic to humans (Group 2B).

Chlorinated drinking-water was evaluated in 1990 (IARC, 1991) and the overall evaluation was that chlorinated drinking-water is not classifiable as to its carcinogenicity to humans (Group 3). Studies with chlorinated drinking-water gave no evidence for carcinogenicity of chloroform in humans (Group 3) (IARC, 1991).

A drinking-water guideline value of 200 μg/litre for an excess lifetime cancer risk of 10^{-5} has been recommended for chloroform by the World Health Organization (WHO, 1993).

REFERENCES

Abdel-Rahman HS (1982) The presence of trihalomethanes in soft drinks. J Appl Toxicol, 2: 165-166.

Abernethy S, Bobra AM, Shiu WY, Wells PG, & Mackay D (1986) Acute lethal toxicity of hydrocarbons and chlorinated hydrocarbons to two planktonic crustaceans: the key role of organism-water partitioning. Aquat Toxicol, 8: 163-174.

Adriani J (1970) The pharmacology of anaesthetic drugs. Springfield, Illinois, Charles C. Thomas, pp 57-60.

Aggazzotti G, Predieri G, Fantuzzi G, & Benedetti A (1987) Headspace gas chromatographic analysis for determining low levels of chloroform in human plasma. J Chromatogr, 416: 125-130.

Aggazzotti G, Fantuzzi G, Tartoni PL, & Predieri G (1990) Plasma chloroform concentrations in swimmers using indoor swimming pools. Arch Environ Health, 45(3): 175-179.

Agustin JS & Lim-Sylianco CY (1978) Mutagenic and clastogenic effects of chloroform. Bull Phil Biochem Sci, 1: 17-23.

Ahmadizadeh M, Echt R, Kuo C-H, & Hook JB (1984) Sex and strain differences in mouse kidney: Bowman's capsule morphology and susceptibility to chloroform. Toxicol Lett, 20: 161-172.

Ahmed AF, Kubic VL, & Anders MW (1977) Metabolism of haloforms to carbon monoxide: I. *In vitro* studies. Drug Metab Dispos, 5: 198-204.

Allard U & Andersson L (1992) Exposure of dental personnel to chloroform in root filling procedures. Endod Dent Traumatol, 8: 155-159.

Althaus FR, Lawrence SD, Sattler GL, Longfellow DG, & Pitot HC (1982) Chemical quantification of unscheduled DNA synthesis in cultured hepatocytes as an assay for the rapid screening of potential chemical carcinogens. Cancer Res, 42: 3010-3015.

Anderson DR & Lusty EW (1980) Acute toxicity and bioaccumulation of chloroform to 4 species of freshwater fish. Richland, WA, Battelle Pacific North West Laboratory (NUREG/CR-0893).

Appleby A, Kazazis J, Lillian D, & Singh HB (1976) Atmospheric formation of chloroform from trichloroethylene. J Environ Sci Health, A11: 711-715.

Armstrong DW & Golden T (1986) Determination of distribution and concentration of trihalomethanes in aquatic recreational and therapeutic facilities by electron capture GC. LC-GC, 4: 652-655.

Athanasiou K & Kyrtopoulos SA (1981) Induction of sister chromatid exchange by non-mutagenic carcinogens. NATO Adv Study Inst Ser A, 40: 557-562.

ATSDR (1993) Toxicological profile for chloroform (update). Atlanta, Georgia, Agency for Toxic Substances and Disease Registry.

Azri-Meehan S, Mata MP, Gandafi AJ, & Brendel K (1992) The hepatotoxicity of chloroform in precision-cut rat liver slices. Toxicology, 73: 239-250.

Bai C-L, Canfield PJ, & Stacey NH (1992) Individual serum bile acids as early indicators of carbon tetrachloride- and chloroform-induced liver injury. Toxicology, 75: 221-234.

Baker SU & Bonin AM (1981) Study of 42 coded compounds with the Salmonella/mammalian microsome assay. In: De Serres FJ & Ashby J ed. Evaluation of short-term tests for carcinogens: Report of the international collaborative study. Amsterdam, Oxford, New York, Elsevier North/Holland, pp 249-260 (Progress in Mutation Research, Volume 1).

Balster RL & Borzelleca JF (1982) Behavioural toxicity of trihalomethane contaminants of drinking water in mice. Environ Health Perspect, 46: 127-136.

Bätjer K, Cetinkaya M, Düszeln v J, Gabel B, Lahl U, Stachel B, & Thiemann W (1980) Chloroform emission into urban atmosphere. Chemosphere, 9: 311-316.

Bauer U (1981) [Human exposure to environmental chemicals - Investigations on volatile organic halogenated compounds in water, air, food and human tissues. III. Communication: Results of investigations.] Zbl Bakt Hyg, 1. Abt Orig, B174: 200-237 [in German].

Baumann OE, Drangsholt H, & Carlberg GE (1981) Analysis of volatile halogenated organic compounds in fish. Sci Total Environ, 20: 205-215.

Benoit FM & Jackson R (1987) Trihalomethane formation in whirlpool spas. Water Res, 2: 353-357.

Bergman K (1984) Application and results of whole-body autoradiography in distribution studies of organic solvents. Crit Rev Toxicol, 12: 59-119.

Birge WJ (1980) Effects of organic compounds on amphibian reproduction. Lexington, University of Kentucky, Water Resources Research Institute (Research Report No. 121; PB80-147523).

Birge WJ, Black JA & Bruser DM (1979) Toxicity of organic chemicals to embryo-larval stages of fish. Washington, DC, Environmental Protection Agency (EPA-560/11-79-007; PB80-101637).

Blancato JN & Chiu (1994) Use of pharmacokinetic models to estimate internal doses from exposure. In: Wang R ed. Water contamination and health. New York, Marcel Dekker, Inc.

Bogen KT, Colston BW, & Machicao LK (1992) Dermal absorption of dilute aqueous chloroform, trichloroethylene, and tetrachloroethylene in hairless guinea pigs. Fundam Appl Toxicol, 18: 30-39.

Bomski HA, Sobdewska A, & Strakowski A (1967) [Toxic damage of the liver by chloroform in chemical industry workers.] Int Arch Gewerbepathol Gewerbehyg, 24: 127-134 [in German]

Borzelleca JF & Carchman RA (1982) Effect of selected organic drinking water contaminants on male reproduction. Research Triangle Park, North Carolina, US Environmental Protection Agency (EPA 600/-/1-82-009; PB82-259847).

Bouwer EJ & McCarty PL (1983) Transformation of 1- and 2-carbon halogenated aliphatic organic compounds under methanogenic conditions. Appl Environ Microbiol, **45**: 1286-1294.

Bouwer EJ, Rittmann BE, & McCarty PL (1981) Anaerobic degradation of halogenated 1- and 2-carbon organic compounds. Environ Sci Technol, **15**: 596-599.

Bowman FJ, Borzelleca JF, & Munson AE (1978) The toxicity of some halomethanes in mice. Toxicol Appl Pharmacol, **44**: 213-215.

Brady JF, Li D, Ishizaki H, Lee M, Ning SM, Xiao F, & Yang CS (1989) Induction of cytochromes P450IIE1 and P450IIB1 by secondary ketones and the role of P450IIE1 in chloroform metabolism. Toxicol Appl Pharmacol, **100**: 342-349.

Branchflower RV, Schulick RD, George JW, & Pohl LR (1983) Comparison of the effects of methyl *n*-butyl ketone and phenobarbital on rat liver cytochrome P-450 and the metabolism of chloroform to phosgene. Toxicol Appl Pharmacol, **71**: 414-421.

Brass JH, Feige MA, & Halloran T (1977) The national organic monitoring survey: sampling and analyses of purgeable organic compounds. In: Drinking water quality enhancement source protection, pp 393-416.

Bringmann G (1973) [Determination of the harmful biological effect of water pollutants from the inhibition of glucose assimilation in the bacterium *Pseudomonas fluorescens*.] Gesund-Ing, **94**: 366-369 (in German).

Bringmann G (1975) [Determination of the harmful biological effect of water pollutants from the inhibition of cell reproduction in the blue alga *Microcystis*.] Gesund-Ing, **96**: 238-241 (in German).

Bringmann G (1978) [Determination of the harmful biological effect of water pollutants on protozoa. I. Bacteriophagic flagellates.] Z Wasser-Abwasser Forsch, **11**: 210-215 (in German).

Bringmann G & Kühn R (1977) [Threshold values for the harmful effect of water pollutants on bacteria (*Pseudomonas putida*) and green algae (*Scenedesmus quadricauda*) in the cell reproduction inhibition test.] Z Wasser-Abwasser Forsch, **10**: 87-97 (in German).

Bringmann G & Kühn R (1980) [Determination of the harmful biological effect of water pollutants on protozoa. II. Bacteriophagic ciliates.] Z Wasser-Abwasser Forsch, **13**: 26-31 (in German).

Bringmann G, Kühn R, & Winter A (1980) [Determination of the harmful biological effect of water pollutants on protozoa. III. Saprozoic flagellates.] Z Wasser-Abwasser Forsch, **13**: 170-173 (in German).

Brondeau MT, Bonnet P, Guenier JP, & De Ceaurriz J (1983) Short-term inhalation test for evaluating industrial hepatotoxicants in rats. Toxicol Lett, **19**: 139-146.

Brooks TM & Dean BJ (1981) Mutagenic activity of 42 coded compounds in the Salmonella/microsome assay with preincubation. In: De Serres FJ & Ashby J ed. Evaluation of short-term tests for carcinogens: Report of the international collaborative study. Amsterdam, Oxford, New York, Elsevier North/Holland, pp 261-270 (Progress in Mutation Research, Volume 1).

Brown BR Jr (1972) Hepatic microsomal lipoperoxidation and inhalation anaesthetics: A biochemical and morphologic study in the rat. Anesthesiology, 36: 458-465.

Brown BR, Sipes IG, & Sagalyn AM (1974a) Mechanisms of acute hepatic toxicity: chloroform, halothane and glutathione. Anesthesiology 41: 554-561.

Brown DM, Langley PF, Smith D, & Taylor DC (1974b) Metabolism of chloroform. I. The role of [^{14}C]-chloroform by different species. Xenobiotica, 4: 151-163.

Budavari S ed. (1989) The Merck index: an encyclopedia of chemicals, drugs and biologicals, 11th ed. Rahway, New Jersey, Merck and Co.

Bull RJ & Kopfler FC (1991) Health Effects of disinfectants and disinfection by-products. Denver, Colorado, AWWA Research Foundation and American Water Works Association, pp 14, 99-104.

Bull RJ, Brown JM, Meierhenry EA, Jorgenson TA, Robinson M, & Stober JA (1986) Enhancement of the hepatotoxicity of CHCl$_3$ in B6C3F$_1$ mice by corn oil: Implications for CHCl$_3$ carcinogenesis. Environ Health Perspect, 69: 49-58.

Burkhalter JE & Balster RL (1979) Behavioral teratology evaluation of trichloromethane in mice. Neurobehav Toxicol, 1: 199-205.

Butler TC (1961) Reduction of carbon tetrachloride *in vivo* and reduction of carbon tetrachloride and chloroform *in vitro* by tissues and tissue constituents. J Pharmacol Exp Ther, 134: 311-319.

Butterworth BE, Smith-Oliver T, Earle L, Loury DJ, White RD, Doolittle DJ, Working PK, Cattley RC, Jirtle R, Michalopoulos G, & Strom S (1989) Use of primary cultures of human hepatocytes in toxicology studies. Cancer Res, 49: 1075-1084.

Callen DF, Wolf CR, & Philpot RM (1980) Cytochrome P-450 mediated genetic activity and cytotoxicity of seven halogenated aliphatic hydrocarbons in *Saccharomyces cerevisiae*. Mutat Res, 77: 55-63.

Capel ID, Dorrell HM, Jenner M, Pinnock MH, & Williams DC (1979) The effect of chloroform ingestion on the growth of murine tumours. Eur J Cancer, 15: 1485-1490.

Challen PJR, Hickish DE, & Bedford J (1958) Chronic chloroform intoxication. Br J Ind Med, 15: 243-249.

Charbonneau M, Greselin E, Brodeur J, & Plaa GL (1991) Influence of acetone on the severity of the liver injury induced by haloalkane mixtures. Can J Physiol Pharmacol, 69(12): 1901-1907.

Cherkin A & Catchpool JF (1964) Temperature dependence of anesthesia in goldfish. Science, 144: 1460-1462.

Chinery RL & Gleason AK (1993) A compartmental model for prediction of breath concentration and absorbed dose of chloroform after exposure while showering. Risk Anal, 13(1): 51-62.

Chiou WL (1975) Quantitation of hepatic and pulmonary first-pass effect and its implications in pharmacokinetic study. I. Pharmacokinetics of chloroform in man. J Pharmacokinet Biopharm, 3: 193-201.

Chu I, Secours V, Marino I, & Villeneuve DC (1980) The acute toxicity of four trihalomethanes in male and female rats. Toxicol Appl Pharmacol, 52: 351-353.

Chu I, Villeneuve DC, Secours VE, & Becking GC (1982a) Toxicity of trihalomethanes. I. The acute and subacute toxicity of chloroform, bromodichloromethane, chlorodibromomethane and bromoform in rats. J Environ Sci Health, B17: 205-224.

Chu I, Villeneuve DC, Secours VE, & Becking GC (1982b) Toxicity of trihalomethanes. II. Reversibility of toxicological changes produced by chloroform, bromodichloromethane, chlorodibromomethane and bromoform in rats. J Environ Sci Health, B17: 225-240.

Clemens TL, Hill RN, Bullock LP, Johnson WD, Sultatos LG, & Vessel ES (1979) Chloroform toxicity in the mouse: Role of genetic factors and steroids. Toxicol Appl Pharmacol, 48: 117-130.

Cohen EN & Hood N (1969) Application of low-temperature autoradiography to studies of the uptake and metabolism of volatile anaesthetic in the mouse. Anesthesiology, 30: 306-314.

Colacci A, Bartoli S, Bonora B, Guidotti L, Lattanzi G, Mazzullo M, Niero A, Perocco P, Silingardi P, & Grilli S (1991) Chloroform bioactivation leading to nucleic acids binding. Tumori, 77(4): 285-290.

Condie LW, Smallwood CL, & Laurie RD (1983) Comparative renal and hepatotoxicity of halomethanes: bromodichloromethane, bromoform, chloroform, dibromochloromethane and methylene chloride. Drug Chem Toxicol, 6: 563-578.

Conlon MF (1963) Addiction to chlorodyne. Br Med J, 2: 1177-1178.

Corley RA, Mendrala AL, Smith FA, Staats DA, Gargas ML, Conolly RB, Andersen ME, & Reitz RH (1990) Development of a physiologically based pharmacokinetic model for chloroform. Toxicol Appl Pharmacol, 103: 512-527.

Cortés F, Mateos S, & Escalza P (1985) C-Mitosis, chromosomal aberrations and sister chromatid exchanges induced by chloroform in root-tip cells of *Allium cepa*. Cytobios, 44: 231-237.

Cowgill UM, Milazzo DP, & Landenberger BD (1989) Toxicity of nine benchmark chemicals to *Skeletonema costatum*, a marine diatom. Environ Toxicol Chem, 8: 451-455.

Cowlen MS, Hewitt WR, & Schroeder F (1984a) 2-Hexanone potentiation of (14C)chloroform hepatotoxicity: covalent interaction of a reactive intermediate with rat liver phospholipids. Toxicol Appl Pharmacol, 73: 478-491.

Cowlen MS, Hewitt WR, & Schroeder F (1984b) Mechanism in 2-hexanone potentiation of chloroform hepatotoxicity. Toxicol Lett, 22: 293-299.

Cox RA, Derwent RG, Eggleton AEJ, & Lovelock JE (1976) Photochemical oxidation of halocarbons in the troposphere. Atmos Environ, 10: 305-308.

Cresteil TL, Beaune Ph, Leroux JP, Lange M, & Mansuy D (1979) Biotransformation of chloroform by rat and human liver microsomes; *in vitro* effect on some enzyme activities and mechanisms of irreversible binding to macromolecules. Chem-Biol Interact, 24: 153-165.

Cronn DR & Harsch DE (1979) Determination of atmospheric halocarbon concentration by gas chromatographic-mass spectrometry. Anal Lett, 12: 1489-1496.

Culliford D & Hewitt HB (1957) The influence of sex hormone status on the susceptibility of mice to chloroform-induced necrosis of renal tubules. J Endocrinol, 14: 381-393.

Daft JA (1988) Fumigant contamination during large-scale food sampling for analysis. Arch Environ Contam Toxicol, 17: 177-181.

Daft JA (1989) Determination of fumigants and related chemicals in fatty and non-fatty foods. J Agric Food Chem, 37: 560-564.

Daniel MR & Dehnel JM (1981) Cell transformation test with baby hamster kidney cells. In: De Serres FJ & Ashby J ed. Evaluation of short-term tests for carcinogens: Report of the international collaborative study. Amsterdam, Oxford New York, Elsevier North/Holland, pp 626-637 (Progress in Mutation Research, Volume 1).

Daniel FB, De Angelo AB, Stober JA, Pereira MA, & Olson GR (1989) Chloroform inhibition of 1,2-dimethylhydrazine-induced gastrointestinal tract tumours in the Fischer 344 rat. Fundam Appl Toxicol, 13: 40-45.

Daniel FB, Reddy TV, Stober JA, & Olson GR (1991) Site specific modulation of carcinogen-induced gastrointestinal tract nuclear anomalies in B6C3F$_1$ mice by chloroform. Anticancer Res, 11: 665-670.

Danielsson BRG, Ghantous H, & Dencker L (1986) Distribution of chloroform and methyl chloroform and their metabolites in pregnant mice. Biol Res Pregnancy, 7: 77-83.

Davis ME (1992) Dichloroacetic acid and trichloroacetic acid increase chloroform toxicity. J Toxicol Environ Health, 37: 139-148.

Davis ME & Berndt WO (1992) Sex differences in monochloroacetate pretreatment effects on chloroform toxicity in rats. Fundam Appl Toxicol, 18: 66-71.

Davis DD, Machado G, Conaway B, Oh Y, & Watson R (1976) A temperature dependent kinetics study of the reaction of OH with CH_3Cl, CH_2Cl_2, $CHCl_3$ and CH_3Br. J Chem Phys, 65: 1268-1274.

De Biasi A, Sbraccia M, Keizer J, Testai E, & Vittozzi L (1992) The regioselective binding of $CHCl_3$ reactive intermediates to microsomal phospholipids. Chem-Biol Interact, 85: 229-242.

Deml E & Oesterle D (1985) Dose-dependent promoting activity of chloroform in rat liver foci bioassay. Cancer Letters, 29: 59-63.

Deml E & Oesterle D (1987) Dose-response of promotion by polychlorinated biphenyls and chloroform in rat liver foci bioassay. Arch Toxicol, 60: 209-211.

Den Hartog JC (1980, 1981) [Analysis of gaseous organic components in the outdoor air.] Rijswijk, The Netherlands, TNO, Prins Maurits Laboratory (Reports PML-TNO Nos 1980-182, 1981-149, 1981-155, 1981-158((in Dutch).

Deringer MK, Dunn TB, & Heston WE (1953) Results of strain C3H mice to chloroform. Proc Soc Exp Biol Med, 83: 474-479.

De Serres FJ & Ashby J ed. (1981) Evaluation of short-term tests for carcinogens: Report of the international collaborative study. Amsterdam, Oxford, New York, Elsevier North/Holland (Progress in Mutation Research, Volume 1).

Dilling WL (1977) Interphase transfer process. II. Evaporation rates of chloromethanes, ethanes, ethylenes, propanes, and propylenes from dilute aqueous solutions. Comparisons with theoretical predictions. Environ Sci Technol, 11: 405-409.

Dimitriades B, Gay BW Jr, Arnts RR, & Seila RL (1983) Photochemical reactivity of perchloroethylene: a new appraisal. J Air Pollut Control Assoc, 33: 575.

Divincenzo GD & Krasavage WJ (1974) Serum ornithine carbamyl transferase as a liver response test for exposure to organic solvents. Am Ind Hyg Assoc J, 35: 21-29.

Docks EL & Krishna G (1976) The role of glutathione in chloroform induced hepatotoxicity. Exp Mol Pathol, 24: 13-22.

Dowty BJ, Laseter JL, & Storer J (1976) The transplacental migration and accumulation in blood of volatile organic constituents. Pediatr Res, 10: 696-701.

Duprat P, Delsaut L, & Gradiski D (1976) Pouvoir irritant des principaux chlorés aliphatiques sur la peau et les muqueuses oculaires du lapin. Eur J Toxicol Environ Hyg, 9: 171-177.

Ebel RE, Barlow RL, & McGrath EA (1987) Chloroform hepatotoxicity in the Mongolian gerbil. Fundam Appl Toxicol, 8: 207-216.

ECDIN (1992) On-line search in the environmental chemicals data and information network. ECDIN/copyright JRC-CEC/ISPRA.

Egli C, Scholtz R, Cook AM, & Leisinger T (1987) Anaerobic dechlorination of tetrachloromethane and 1,2-dichloroethane to degradable products by pure cultures of *Desulfobacterium* sp. and *Methanobacterium* sp. FEMS Microbiol Lett, 43: 257-261.

Entz RC, Thomas KW, & Diachenko GW (1982) Residues of volatile halocarbons in foods using headspace gas chromatography. J Agric Food Chem, 30: 846-849.

Environment Canada (1986) Ambient air concentration of volatile organic compounds in Toronto and Montreal. Ottawa, Environment Canada, Pollution Measurement Division (Unpublished report).

Environment Canada (1992) Volatile organic compounds measurements in Canadian urban and rural areas: 1989-1991. Ottawa, Environment Canada, Technology Development Branch (Internal report 92-75.16).

Erickson MD (1981) Acquisition and chemical analysis of mother's milk for selected toxic substances. Gov Rep Announc Index US, 5096 (PB81-231029).

Europ-Cost (1976) A comprehensive list of polluting substances which have been identified in various fresh waters, effluent discharges, aquatic animals and plants, and bottom sediments, 2nd ed. Luxembourg, Commission of the European Communities, p 31 (EUCO/MDU/73/76, XII/476/76).

Ewing BB, Chian ESK, & Cook JC (1977) Monitoring to detect previously unrecognized pollutants in surface waters. Appendix: Organic analysis data. Washington, DC, US Environmental Protection Agency (EPA/560/6-77-015).

Federal Office of the Environment (1981) [Clean air '81: development, situation, trends.] Berlin, Federal Office of the Environment (BUA) (in German).

Foster GD & Tullis RE (1985) Quantitative structure-toxicity relationships with osmotically stressed *Artemia salina* nauplii. Environ Pollut, A38: 273-281.

Fry J, Taylor R, & Hathway DE (1972) Pulmonary elimination of chloroform and its metabolite in man. Arch Int Pharmacodyn Ther, 196: 98-111.

Fujie K, Aoki T, & Wada M (1990) Acute and subacute cytogenetic effects of the trihalomethanes on rat bone marrow cells *in vivo*. Mutat Res, 242: 111-119.

Fujie K, Aoki T, & Mae S (1993) Sister-chromatid exchanges induced by trihalomethanes in rat erythroblastic cells. Mutat Res, 300: 241-246.

Garner RC, Welch A, & Pickering C (1981) Mutagenic activity of 42 coded compounds in the Salmonella/microsome assay. In: De Serres FJ & Ashby J ed. Evaluation of short-term tests for carcinogens: Report of the international collaborative study. Amsterdam, Oxford, New York, Elsevier North/Holland, pp 280-284 (Progress in Mutation Research, Volume 1).

Gatehouse D (1981) Mutagenic activity of 42 coded compounds in the "microtiter" fluctuation test. In: De Serres FJ & Ashby J ed. Evaluation of short-term tests for carcinogens: Report of the international collaborative study. Amsterdam, Oxford, New York, Elsevier North/Holland, pp 376-386 (Progress in Mutation Research, Volume 1).

Gearhart JM, Seckel C, & Vinegar A (1993) *In vivo* metabolism of chloroform in B6C3F1, mice determined by the method of gas uptake: the effects of body temperature on tissue partition coefficients and metabolism. Toxicol Appl Pharmacol, 119: 258-266.

Gersich FM, Blanchard FA, Applegath SL, & Park CN (1986) The precision of Daphnid (*Daphnia magna* Straus, 1820) static acute toxicity tests. Arch Environ Contam Toxicol, 15: 741-749.

Glende EA & Recknagel RO (1992) Phosphodipase A_2 activation and cell injury in isolated rat hepatocytes exposed to bromotrichloromethane, chloroform, and 1,1-dichloro-ethylene as compared to effects of carbon tetrachloride. Toxicol Appl Pharmacol, 113: 159-162.

Gocke E, King M-T, Eckhardt K, & Wild D (1981) Mutagenicity of cosmetics ingredients licensed by the European Communities. Mutat Res, 90: 91-109.

Goodman LS & Gilman AG (1970) The pharmacological basis of therapeutics. New York, McMillan Co.

Gradiski D, Magadur JL, Baillot M, Danière MC, & Schuh MB (1974) Toxicité comparée des principaux solvants chlorés aliphatiques. J Eur Toxicol, 7: 247-254.

Gradiski D, Bonnet P, Raoult G, & Magadur JL (1978) Toxicité aiguë comparée par inhalation des principaux solvants aliphatiques chlorés. Arch Mal Prof Méd Trav Sécur Soc, 39: 249-257.

Green MHL (1981) A differential killing test using an improved repair-deficient strain of *Escherichia coli*. In: De Serres FJ & Ashby J ed. Evaluation of short-term tests for carcinogens: Report of the international collaborative study. Amsterdam, Oxford, New York, Elsevier North/Holland, pp 183-194 (Progress in Mutation Research, Volume 1).

Greim H, Bimboe SD, Egert G, Göggelmann W, & Krämer M (1977) Mutagenicity and chromosomal aberrations as an analytical tool for *in vitro* detection of mammalian enzyme-mediated formation of reactive metabolites. Arch Toxicol, 39: 159-169.

Grob K (1984) Further development of direct aqueous injection with electron-capture detection in gas chromatography. J Chromatogr, 299: 1-11.

Groger WKL & Grey TF (1979) Effect of chloroform on the activities of liver enzymes in rats. Toxicology, 14: 23-28.

Gualandi G (1984) Genotoxicity of the free-radical producers CCl_4 and lipoperoxidation in *Aspergillus nidulans*. Mutat Res, 136: 109-114.

Guengerich FP, Kim DH, & Iwasaki M (1991) Role of human cytochrome P450 II E1 in the oxidation of suspected carcinogens. Chem Res Toxicol, 4: 160-179.

Hakim A, Jain AK, & Jain R (1992) Chloroform ingestion causing toxic hepatitis. J Assoc Phys India, 40: 477.

Hamada N & Peterson RE (1977) Effect of chlorinated aliphatic hydrocarbons on excretion of protein and electrolytes by rat pancreas. Toxicol Appl Pharmacol, 39: 185-194.

Hardie DWF (1964) Chlorocarbons and chlorohydrocarbons. Chloroform. In: Kirk RE & Othmer DF ed. Encyclopedia of chemical technology, 2nd ed. Vol 5, pp 119-127.

Harms MS, Peterson RE, Fujimoto JM, & Erwin CP (1976) Increased "bile duct-pancreatic fluid" flow in chlorinated hydrocarbon-treated rats. Toxicol Appl Pharmacol, 35: 41-49.

Harris RN, Ratnayake JH, Garry VF, & Anders MW (1982) Interactive hepatotoxicity of chloroform and carbon tetrachloride. Toxicol Appl Pharmacol, 63: 281-289.

Harsch DE & Cronn DR (1978) Low-pressure sample-transfer technique for analysis of stratospheric air samples. J Chromatogr Sci, 16: 363-367.

Hatch GC, Mamay DD, Ayer ML, Casto BC, & Nesnow S (1983) Chemical enhancement of viral transformation in Syrian hamster embryo cells by gaseous and volatile chlorinated methanes and ethanes. Cancer Res, 43: 1945-1950.

Heil E, Oeser H, Hatz R, & Kelker H (1979) [Gas-chromatographic determination of traces of C_1- and C_2- fluoro- and chlorohydrocarbons in air.] Fresenius Z Anal Chem, 297: 357-364 (in German).

Heilbrunn G, Liebert E, & Szanto PB (1945) Chronic chloroform poisoning. Arch Neurol Psychiatr, 53: 68-72.

Herren-Freund SL & Pereira MA (1986) Carcinogenicity of by-products of disinfection in mouse and in rat liver. Environ Health Perspect, 69: 59-66.

Hertlein F (1980) Monitoring airborne contaminants in chemical laboratories. ACS Symp Ser, **120**: 215-230.

Herzfeld D, Van der Gun KD, & Louw R (1989) Quantitative determination of volatile organochlorine compounds in water by GC-headspace analysis with dibromomethane as an internal standard. Chemosphere, **18**: 1425-1430.

Hewitt HB (1956) Renal necrosis in mice after accidental exposure to chloroform. Br J Exp Pathol, **37**: 32-39.

Hewitt WR, Miyajima H, Côté MG, & Plaa GL (1979) Acute alteration of chloroform-induced hepato- and nephrotoxicity by mirex and kepone. Toxicol Appl Pharmacol, **48**: 509-527.

Hewitt WR, Brown EM, Côté MG, Plaa GL, & Miyajima H (1982) Alteration of chloroform-induced nephrotoxicity by exogenous ketones. In: Porter G ed. Nephrotoxic mechanisms of drugs and environmental toxins. New York, London, Plenum, Press, pp 357-365.

Hewitt LA, Palmason C, Masson S, & Plaa GL (1990) Evidence for the involvement of organelles in the mechanism of ketone-potentiated chloroform-induced hepatotoxicity. Liver, **10**: 35-48.

Heywood R, Sortwell RJ, Noel PRB, Street AE, Prentice DE, Roe FJC, Wardsworth PF, Worden AN, & Van Abbé NJ (1979) Safety evaluation of toothpaste containing chloroform. III. Long-term study in beagle dogs. J Environ Pathol Toxicol, **2**: 835-851.

Hill RN (1978) Differential toxicity of chloroform in the mouse. Ann NY Acad Sci, **298**: 170-175.

Hill RN, Clemens TL, Liu DK, Vesell ES, & Johnson WD (1975) Genetic control of chloroform toxicity in mice. Science, **190**: 159-160.

Howard Carleton J & Evenson KM (1976) Rate constants for the reactions of OH with CH_4 and fluorine, chlorine and bromine substituted methanes at 296 K. J Chem Phys, **64**: 197.

Hubbard SA, Green MHL, Bridges BA, Wain AJ, & Bridges JW (1981) Fluctuation test with S_9 and hepatocyte activation. In: De Serres FJ & Ashby J ed. Evaluation of short-term tests for carcinogens: Report of the international collaborative study. Amsterdam, Oxford, New York, Elsevier North/Holland, pp 361-370 (Progress in Mutation Research, Volume 1).

IARC (1979) Chloroform. In: Some halogenated hydrocarbons. Lyon, International Agency for Research on Cancer, pp 401-427 (IARC Monographs on the Evaluation of the Carcinogenic Risk of Chemicals to Humans, Volume 20).

IARC (1987) Overall evaluations of carcinogenicity: An updating of IARC monographs volumes 1 to 42. Lyon, International Agency for Research on Cancer, pp 152-154 (IARC Monographs on the Evaluation of the Carcinogenic Risk of Chemicals to Humans, Supplement 7).

IARC (1991) Chlorinated drinking-water. In: Chlorinated drinking-water; chlorination by-products; some other halogenated compounds; cobalt and cobalt compounds. Lyon, International Agency for Research on Cancer, pp 45-141 (IARC Monographs on the Evaluation of Carcinogenic Risks to Humans, Volume 52).

Ichinotsubo D, Mower H, & Mandel M (1981a) Testing of a series of paired compounds (carcinogen and non-carcinogenic structural analog) by DNA repair-deficient *E. coli* strains. In: De Serres FJ & Ashby J ed. Evaluation of short-term tests for carcinogens: Report of the international collaborative study. Amsterdam, Oxford, New York, Elsevier North/Holland, pp 195-198 (Progress in Mutation Research, Volume 1).

Ichinotsubo D, Mower H, & Mandel M (1981b) Mutagen testing of a series of paired compounds with the Ames Salmonella testing system. In: De Serres FJ & Ashby J eds. Evaluation of short-term tests for carcinogens: Report of the international collaborative study. Amsterdam, Oxford, New York, Elsevier North/Holland, pp 298-301 (Progress in Mutation Research, Volume 1).

Iijima M, Côté MG, & Plaa GL (1983) A semiquantitative morphologic assessment of chlordecone-potentiated chloroform hepatotoxicity. Toxicol Lett, 17: 307-314.

Ikatsu H & Nakajima T (1992) Hepatotoxic interaction between carbon tetrachloride and chloroform in ethanol treated rats. Arch Toxicol, 66: 580-586.

Ilett KF, Reid WD, Sipes IG, & Krishna G (1973) Chloroform toxicity in mice: correlation of renal and hepatic necrosis with covalent binding of metabolites to tissue macromolecules. Exp Mol Pathol, 19: 215-229.

Jagannath DR, Vultaggio DM, & Brusick DJ (1981) Genetic activity of 42 coded compounds in the mitotic gene conversion assay using *Saccharomyces cerevisiae* strain D4. In: De Serres FJ & Ashby J ed. Evaluation of short-term tests for carcinogens: Report of the international collaborative study. Amsterdam, Oxford, New York, Elsevier North/Holland, pp 456-467 (Progress in Mutation Research, Volume 1).

Jo WK, Weisel CP, & Lioy PJ (1990a) Routes of chloroform exposure and body burden from showering with chlorinated tap water. Risk Anal, 10: 575-580.

Jo WK, Weisel CP, & Lioy PJ (1990b) Chloroform exposure and the health risk associated with multiple uses of chlorinated tap water. Risk Anal, 10: 581-585.

Jones JRE (1947) The oxygen consumption of *Gasterosteus aculeatus* in toxic solutions. Exp Biol, 23: 298-311.

Jones WM, Margolis G, & Stephen CR (1958) Hepatotoxicity of inhalation anaesthetic drugs. Anesthesiology, 19: 715-723.

Jorgenson TA, Meierhenry EF, Rushbrook CJ, Bull RJ, & Robinson M (1985) Carcinogenicity of chloroform in drinking water to male Osborne-Mendel rats and female B6C3F1 mice. Fundam Appl Toxicol, 5: 760-769.

Jorgenson TA & Rushbrook CJ (1980) Effects of chloroform in the drinking water of rats and mice. Ninety-day subacute toxicity study. Washington, DC, US Environmental Protection Agency (EPA-600/1-80-030; NTIS PB80-219108).

Jorgenson TA, Rushbrook CJ, & Jones DCL (1982) Dose-response study of chloroform carcinogenesis in the mouse and rat: status report. Environ Health Perspect, 46: 141-149.

Juhnke I & Lüdemann D (1978) [Results of the testing of 200 chemical compounds for acute toxicity for fish by means of the golden orfe test.] Z Wasser-Abwasser Forsch, 11: 161-164 (in German).

Kada T (1981) The DNA-damaging activity of 42 coded compounds in the Rec-assay. In: De Serres FJ & Ashby J ed. Evaluation of short-term tests for carcinogens: Report of the international collaborative study. Amsterdam, Oxford, New York, Elsevier North/Holland, pp 175-182 (Progress in Mutation Research, Volume 1).

Kajino M (1977) [Formation of chloroform during chlorination of drinking water.] Chem Abstr, **88**, 27631K (in Japanese).

Kassinova GV, Kovaltsova SV, Marfin SV, & Zakharov IA (1981) Activity of 40 coded compounds in differential inhibition and mitotic crossing-over assays in yeast. In: De Serres FJ & Ashby J ed. Evaluation of short-term tests for carcinogens: Report of the international collaborative study. Amsterdam, Oxford, New York, Elsevier North/Holland, pp 434-455 (Progress in Mutation Research, Volume 1).

Kawamura K & Kaplan IR (1983) Notes: Organic compounds in the rainwater of Los Angeles. Environ Sci Technol, **17**: 497-501.

Kebbekus BB & Bozzelli JW (1982) Determination of selected toxic organic vapours in air by adsorbent trapping and capillary GC. J Environ Sci Health, **A17**: 713-723.

Kedderis GL, Held SD, Pearson AC, & Carfagns MA (1993a) Isolated mouse hepatocytes as an *in vitro* model for the *in vivo* metabolism and cytolethality of chloroform (CF). Toxicologist, **13**: 198.

Kedderis GL, Carfagna MA, Held SD, Batra R, Murphy JE, & Gargas ML (1993b) Kinetic analysis of furan biotransformation by F-344 rats *in vivo* and *in vitro*. Toxicol Appl Pharmacol, **123**: 274-282.

Kerfoot HB (1987) Shallow-probe soil-gas sampling for indication of ground-water contamination by chloroform. Int J Environ Anal Chem, **30**: 167-181.

Kimura ET, Ebert DM, & Dodge PW (1971) Acute toxicity and limits of solvent residue for sixteen organic solvents. Toxicol Appl Pharmacol, **19**: 699-704.

Kirkland DJ, Smith KL, & Van Abbé NJ (1981) Failure of chloroform to induce chromosome damage or sister-chromatid exchange in cultured human lymphocytes and failure to induce reversion in *Escherichia coli*. Food Cosmet Toxicol, **19**: 651-656.

Klaassen CD & Plaa GL (1967) Relative effects of various chlorinated hydrocarbons on liver and kidney in dogs. Toxicol Appl Pharmacol, **10**: 119-131.

Klaassen CD & Plaa GL (1969) Comparison of the biochemical alterations elicited in livers from rats treated with carbon tetrachloride, chloroform, 1,1,2-trichloroethane and 1,1,1-trichloroethane. Biochem Pharmacol, **18**: 2019-2027.

Klaunig JE, Ruch RJ, & Pereira MA (1986) Carcinogenicity of chlorinated methane and ethane compounds administered in drinking water to mice. Environ Health Perspect, **69**: 89-95.

Kluwe WM (1981) The nephrotoxicity of low molecular weight halogenated alkane solvents, pesticides and chemical intermediates. In: Hook JB ed. Toxicology of the kidney. New York, Raven Press Ltd, pp 179-226.

Knie J, Hälke A, Juhnke I, & Schiller W (1983) [Results of studies on chemical substances with four biotests.] Dtsch Gewässerkd Mitt, 27: 77-79 (in German).

Könemann H (1981) Quantitative structure-activity relationships in fish toxicity studies. Part 1: Relationships for 50 industrial pollutants. Toxicology, 19: 209-211.

Koop DR, Morgan ET, Tarr GE, & Coon MJ (1982) Purification and characterization of a unique isozyme of cytochrome P450 from liver microsomes of ethanol-treated rabbits. J Biol Chem, 257: 8472-8480.

Kramer MD, Lynch CF, Isacson P, & Hanson JW (1992) The association of waterborne chloroform with intrauterine growth retardation. Epidemiology, 3: 407-413.

Krasner SW, McGuire MJ, Jacangelo JG, Patania NL, Reagan KM, & Aieta EM (1989) The occurrence of disinfection by-products in U.S. drinking water. J Am Water Works Assoc, 81: 41-53.

Kroneld R (1985) Recovery and reproducibility in determination of volatile halocarbons in water and blood. Bull Environ Contam Toxicol, 34: 486-496.

Krost KJ, Pellizzari ED, Walburn SG, & Hubbard SA (1982) Collection and analysis of hazardous organic emissions. Anal Chem, 54: 810-817.

Kutob SD & Plaa GL (1962a) A procedure of estimating the hepatotoxic potential of certain industrial solvents. Toxicol Appl Pharmacol, 4: 354-361.

Kutob SD & Plaa GL (1962b) The effect of acute ethanol intoxication on chloroform-induced liver damage. J Pharmacol Exp Teratol, 135: 245-251.

Kylin B, Reichard H, Sümegi I, & Yllner S (1963) Hepatotoxicity of inhaled trichloroethylene, tetrachloroethylene and chloroform. Single exposure. Acta Pharmacol Toxicol, 20: 16-26.

Lahl U, Bätjer K, Düszeln v J, Gabel B, Stachel B, & Thiemann W (1981a) Distribution and balance of volatile halogenated hydrocarbons in the water and air of covered swimming pools using chlorine for water disinfection. Water Res, 15: 803-814.

Land PC, Owen EL, & Linde HW (1981) Morphologic changes in mouse spermatozoa after exposure to inhalational anaesthetics during early spermatogenesis. Anesthesiology, 54: 53-56.

Larson JL, Wolf DC, & Butterworth BE (1993) The acute hepatotoxicity and nephrotoxic effects of chloroform in male F-344 rats and female B6C3F$_1$ mice. Fundam Appl Toxicol 20: 302-315.

Larson JL, Wolf DC, & Butterworth BE (1994a) Induced cytotoxicity and cell proliferation in the hepatocarcinogenicity of chloroform in female B6C3F$_1$ mice. Comparison of administration by gavage in corn oil vs ad libitum in drinking water. Fundam Appl Toxicol, 22: 90-102.

Larson JL, Wolf DC, Morgan KT, Méry S, & Butterworth BE, (1994b) The toxicity of one week exposures to inhaled chloroform in female B6C3F$_1$ mice and male F-344 rats. Fundam Appl Toxicol, 22: 431-446.

Larson JL, Sprankle CS, & Butterworth BE (1994c) Lack of chloroform-induced DNA repair *in vitro* and *in vivo* in hepatocytes of female B6C3F$_1$ mice. Environ Mol Mutagen, **23**: 132-136.

Lasa J & Rosiek J (1979) [Detection of halogen compounds in air with a colometric ECD.] Chem Anal, **24**: 819-826 (in Polish).

Lavigne JG & Marchand C (1974) The role of metabolism in chloroform hepatocytotoxicity. Toxicol Appl Pharmacol, **29**: 312-326.

Lavigne JG, Belanger PM, Dore F, & Labrecque G (1983) Temporal variations in chloroform-induced hepatotoxicity in rats. Toxicology, **26**: 267-273.

LeBlanc GA (1980) Acute toxicity of priority pollutants to water flea (*Daphnia magna*). Bull Environ Contam Toxicol, **24**: 684-691.

Lehmann KB & Flury FF (1943) Chlorinated hydrocarbons. In: Lehmann KB & Flury FF ed. Toxicology and hygiene of industrial solvents. Baltimore, Maryland, Williams & Wilkins Co, pp 138-145, 191-196.

Lehmann KB & Hasegawa (1910) [Study on the absorption of chlorinated hydrocarbons from the air by animal and man.] Arch Hyg, **72**: 327-342 (in German).

Leveson R & Barker N (1981) Airscan: an ultrasensitive trace air impurity analyzer for use in toxic aviation environments (AGARD Conf Proc AGARD-CP-309, B15/1-B15/12).

Lillian D & Singh HB (1974) Absolute determination of atmospheric halocarbons by gas phase coulometry. Anal Chem, **46**: 1060-1063.

Linde HW & Mesnick PS (1979) Causes of death of anaesthesiologists from the chloroform era. Washington, DC, US Environmental Protection Agency (EPA 600/1-179-043; NTIS PB80-125172).

Lioy PJ & Lioy MJ ed. (1983) Air sampling instruments for evaluation of atmospheric contaminants, 6th ed. Cincinnati, Ohio, American Conference of Governmental Industrial Hygienists, pp V/85-V/86.

Löfberg B & Tjälve H (1986) Tracing tissues with chloroform-metabolizing capacity in rats. Toxicology, **39**: 13-35.

Loprieno N (1981) Screening of coded carcinogenic/non carcinogenic chemicals by a forward-mutation system with the yeast *Schizosaccharomyces pombe*. In: De Serres FJ & Ashby J ed. Evaluation of short-term tests for carcinogens: Report of the international collaborative study. Amsterdam, Oxford, New York, Elsevier North/Holland, pp 424-425 (Progress in Mutation Research, Volume 1).

Lundberg I, Ekdahl M, Kronevi T, Lidums V, & Lundberg S (1986) Relative hepatotoxicity of some industrial solvents after intraperitoneal injection or inhalation exposure in rats. Environ Res, **40**: 411-420.

Lurker PA, Clark CS, Elia VJ, Gartside PS, & Kinman RN (1983) Worker exposure to chlorinated organic compounds from the activated sludge wastewater treatment process. Am Ind Hyg Assoc J, **44**: 109-112.

Lyman WJ, Reehl WF, & Rosenblatt DH (1982) Handbook of chemical property estimation methods. New York, McGraw-Hill Book Company.

McConnell G, Ferguson DM, & Pearson CR (1975) Chlorinated hydrocarbons and the environment. Endeavor, 34: 13-18.

MacDonald DJ (1981) Salmonella/microsome tests on 42 coded chemicals. In: De Serres FJ & Ashby J ed. Evaluation of short-term tests for carcinogens: Report of the international collaborative study. Amsterdam, Oxford, New York, Elsevier North/Holland, pp 285-297 (Progress in Mutation Research, Volume 1).

McLean AEM (1970) The effect of protein deficiency and microsomal enzyme induction by DDT and phenobarbitone on the acute toxicity of chloroform and a pyrrolizidine alkaloid, retrorsine. Br J Exp Pathol, 511: 317-321.

McMartin DN, O'Connor JA, & Kaminsky LS (1981) Effects of differential changes in rat hepatic and renal cytochrome P-450 concentrations on hepatotoxicity and nephrotoxicity of chloroform. Res Commun Chem Pathol Pharmacol, 31: 99-110.

Mansuy D, Beaune P, Cresteil T, Lange M, & Leroux JP (1977) Evidence for phosgene formation during liver microsomal oxidation of chloroform. Biochem Biophys Res Commun, 79: 513-517.

Martin CN & McDermid AC (1981) Testing of 42 coded compounds for their ability to induce unscheduled DNA repair synthesis in HeLa cells. In: De Serres FJ & Ashby J ed. Evaluation of short-term tests for carcinogens: Report of the international collaborative study. Amsterdam, Oxford, New York, Elsevier North/Holland, pp 533-537 (Progress in Mutation Research, Volume 1).

Masuda Y, Yano I, & Murano T (1980) Comparative studies on the hepatotoxic actions of chloroform and related halogenomethanes in normal and phenobarbital-pretreated animals. J Pharmacobio-Dyn, 3: 53-64

Matsushima T, Takamoto Y, Shirai A, Sawamura M, & Sugimura T (1981) Reverse mutation test on 42 coded compounds with the *E. coli* WP2 system. In: De Serres FJ & Ashby J ed. Evaluation of short-term tests for carcinogens: Report of the international collaborative study. Amsterdam, Oxford, New York, Elsevier North/Holland, pp 387-395 (Progress in Mutation Research, Volume 1).

Mattice JS, Tsai SC, & Burch MB (1981) Toxicity of trihalomethanes to common carp embryos. Trans Am Fish Soc, 110: 261-269.

Maxwell MI, Burmaster DE, & Ozonoff D (1991) Trihalomethanes. Maximum contaminant levels: the significance of inhalation, dermal exposures to chloroform in household water. Regul Toxicol Pharmacol, 14: 297-312.

Mayes MA, Alexander HC, & Dill DC (1983) A study to assess the influence of age on the response of Fathead minnows in static acute toxicity tests. Bull Environ Contam Toxicol, 31: 139-147.

Mehran MF, Slifker RA, & Cooper WJ (1984) A simplified liquid-liquid extraction method for analysis of trihalomethanes in drinking water. J Chromatogr Sci, 22: 241-243.

Mehta RD & Von Borstel RV (1981) Mutagenic activity of 42 encoded compounds in the haploid yeast reversion assay, strain XV185-14C. In: De Serres FJ & Ashby J ed. Evaluation of short-term tests for carcinogens: Report of the international collaborative study. Amsterdam, Oxford, New York, Elsevier North/Holland, pp 414-423 (Progress in Mutation Research, Volume 1).

Meier JR, Ringhand HP, Coleman WE, Munch JW, Streicher RP, Kaylor WH, & Schenck KM (1985) Identification of mutagenic compounds formed during chlorination of humic acid. Mutat Res, 157: 111-122.

Méry S, Larson JL, Butterworth BE, Wolf DC, Harden R, & Morgan KT (1994) Nasal toxicity of chloroform in male F-344 rats and female B6C3F, mice following a one week inhalation exposure. Toxicol Appl Pharmacol, 125: 214-227.

Mink FL, Coleman WE, Munch JW, Kaylor WH, & Ringhand HP (1983) *In vivo* formation of halogenated reaction products following peroral sodium hypochlorite. Bull Environ Contam Toxicol, 30: 394-399.

Mink FL, Brown TJ, & Rickabaugh J (1986) Absorption, distribution, and excretion of ^{14}C-trihalomethanes in mice and rats. Bull Environ Contam Toxicol, 37: 752-758.

Mirsalis JC, Tyson CK, & Butterworth BE (1982) Detection of genotoxic carcinogens in the *in vivo-in vitro* hepatocyte DNA repair assay. Environ Mutagen, 4: 553-562.

Moore L (1980) Inhibition of liver-microsome calcium pump by *in vivo* administration of CCl_4, $CHCl_3$ and 1,1-dichloroethylene. Biochem Pharmacol, 29: 2505-2511.

Moore DH, Chasseaud LF, Majeed SK, Prentice DE, Roe FJC, & Van Abbé NJ (1982) The effect of dose and vehicle on early tissue damage and regenerative activity after chloroform administration to mice. Food Chem Toxicol, 20: 951-954.

Morele Y, Lefevre C, Ferrari P, Guenier JP, & Muller J (1989) Sampling and analysis of airborne chlorinated methanes - comparison of FID and ECD. Chromatographia, 28: 617-619.

Morgan A, Black A, & Belcher DR (1970) The excretion in breath of some aliphatic halogenated hydrocarbons following administration by inhalation. Ann Occup Hyg, 13: 219-233.

Morgan DL, Cooper SW, Carlock DL, Sykora JJ, Sutton B, Mattie DR, & McDougal JN (1991) Dermal absorption of neat and aqueous volatile organic chemicals in the Fischer-344 rat. Environ Res, 55: 51-63.

Morimoto K & Koizumi A (1983) Trihalomethanes induce sister chromatid exchanges in human lymphocytes *in vitro* and mouse bone marrow cells *in vivo*. Environ Res, 32: 72-79.

Morris RD, Audet AM, Angelillo IF, Chalmers TC, & Mosteller F (1992) Chlorination, chlorination by-products and cancer. A meta-analysis. Am J Public Health, 82: 955.

Munson AE, Sain LE, Sanders VM, Kauffmann BM, White KL, Page DG, Barnes DW, & Borzelleca JF (1982) Toxicology of organic drinking water contaminants: trichloromethane, bromodichloromethane, dibromomethane and tribromomethane. Environ Health Perspect, 46: 117-126.

Murray FJ, Schwetz BA, McBride JF, & Staples RE (1979) Toxicity of inhaled chloroform in pregnant mice and their offspring. Toxicol Appl Pharmacol, 50: 515-522.

Nagao M & Takahashi Y (1981) Mutagenic activity of 42 coded compounds in the Salmonella/microsome assay. In: De Serres FJ & Ashby J ed. Evaluation of short-term tests for carcinogens: Report of the international collaborative study. Amsterdam, Oxford, New York, Elsevier North/Holland, pp 302-313 (Progress in Mutation Research, Volume 1).

Nakajima T & Sato A (1979) Enhanced activity of liver drug-metabolising enzymes for aromatic and chlorinated hydrocarbons following food deprivation. Toxicol Appl Pharmacol, 50: 549-556.

Nakajima T, Koyama Y, & Sato A (1982) Dietary modification of metabolism and toxicity of chemical substances with specific reference to carbohydrate. Biochem Pharmacol, 31: 1005-1011.

Nakajima T, Elovaara E, Park SS, Gelboin HV, & Vainio H (1991) Immunochemical detection of cytochrome P450 isozymes induced in rat liver by n-hexane, 2-hexanone and acetonyl acetone. Arch Toxicol, 65: 542-547.

National Cancer Institute (1976a) Carcinogenesis bioassay of chloroform. Bethesda, Maryland, National Cancer Institute (NTIS PB-264018/AS).

National Cancer Institute (1976b) Report on carcinogenesis bioassay of chloroform. Bethesda, Maryland, National Cancer Institute (NTIS PB-264-018).

Nicloux MM (1906) Passage du chloroforme de la mère au foetus. C R Soc Biol, 60: 373-375.

NNI (Dutch Standardisation Institute) (1984) [Air quality - Outdoor air. Determination of chlorinated hydrocarbons - Coal adsorption/liquid desorption/GC-method.] Dutch Standardisation Institute (Standard NVN 2794) (in Dutch).

Oettel H (1936) [Effects of organic fluids on the skin.] Arch Exp Pathol Pharmacol, 183: 641-696 (in German).

O'Hara TM, Sheppard MA, Clarke EC, Borzelleca JF, Gennings C, & Condie LW (1991) A $CCl_4/CHCl_3$ interaction study in isolated hepatocytes: non-induced and phenobarbital-pretreated cells. J Appl Toxicol, 11: 147-154.

Ohio River Valley Water Sanitation Commission (1980) Assessment of water quality conditions. Ohio River mainstream 1978-79. Cincinnati, Ohio, Ohio River Valley Water Sanitation Commission.

Ohio River Valley Water Sanitation Commission (1982) Assessment of water quality conditions Ohio River mainstream 1980-81. Cincinnati, Ohio, Ohio River Valley Water Sanitation Commission.

Oliver BG (1983) Dihaloacetonitriles in drinking water. Algae and fulvic acid as precursors. Environ Sci Technol, 17: 80-83.

Otson R (1990) A Health and Welfare Canada program to develop personal exposure monitors for airborne organics at $\mu g/m^3$. Proceedings of the 1990 EPA/A & WWMA International Symposium on Measurement of Toxic and Related Air Pollutants (VIP-17). Pittsburg, Pennsylvania, Air & Waste Water Management Association, pp 483-488.

Otson R, Fellin P, & Whitmore R (1992) A national pilot study of airborne VOCs in residences - design and progress. Presented at the 1992 EPA/A & WWMA Symposium on Measurement of Toxic and Related Air Pollutants, Durham, NC, 4-8 May. Pittsburg, Pennsylvania, Air & Waste Water Management Association.

Parry JM & Sharp DC (1981) Induction of mitotic aneuploidy in the yeast strain D6 by 42 coded compounds. In: De Serres FJ & Ashby J ed. Evaluation of short-term tests for carcinogens: Report of the international collaborative study. Amsterdam, Oxford, New York, Elsevier North/Holland, pp 468-480 (Progress in Mutation Research, Volume 1).

Paul BB & Rubinstein D (1963) Metabolism of carbon tetrachloride and chloroform by the rat. J Pharmacol Exp Ther, 141: 141-148.

Pearson CR & McConnell G (1975) Chlorinated C_1 and C_2 hydrocarbons in the marine environment. Proc R Soc Lond, B189: 305-322.

Pellizzari ED, Erickson MD, & Zweidinger (1979) Formulation of preliminary assessment of halogenated organic compounds in man and environmental media. Research Triangle Park, North Carolina, US Environmental Protection Agency (EPA 560/13-79-006).

Pellizzari ED, Hartwell TD, Harris BSH, Waddel RD, Whitaker DA, & Erickson MD (1982) Purgeable organic compounds in mothers' milk. Bull Environ Contam Toxicol, 28: 322-328.

Pellizzari ED, Sheldon LS, & Bursey JT (1985a) Method 25: GC/MS determination of volatile halocarbons in blood and tissue. Environ Carcinog Sel Methods Anal, 7: 435-444.

Pellizzari ED, Zweidinger RA, & Sheldon LS (1985b) Method 24: GC/MS determination of volatile hydrocarbons in breath samples. Environ Carcinog Sel Methods Anal, 7: 413-431.

Pereira MA, Lin L-HC, Lippitt HM, & Herren SL (1982) Trihalomethanes as initiators and promoters of carcinogenesis. Environ Health Perspect, 46: 151-156.

Pereira MA, Knutsen GL, & Herren-Freund SL (1985) Effect of subsequent treatment of chloroform or phenobarbital on the incidence of liver and lung tumours, initiated by ethylnitrosourea in 15 days old mice. Carcinogenesis, 6: 203-207.

Pericin C & Thomann P (1979) Comparison of the acute toxicity of clioquinol, histamine and chloroform in different strains of mice. Arch Toxicol, 2(Suppl): 371-373.

Perocco P & Prodi G (1981) DNA damage by haloalkanes in human lymphocytes cultured in vitro. Cancer Lett, 13: 213-218.

Perocco P, Bolognesi S, & Alberghini W (1983) Toxic activity of seventeen industrial solvents and halogenated compounds on human lymphocytes cultured in vitro. Toxicol Lett, 16: 69-75.

Perry PE & Thomson EJ (1981) Evaluation of the sister chromatid exchange method in mammalian cells as a screening system for carcinogens. In: De Serres FJ & Ashby J ed. Evaluation of short-term tests for carcinogens: Report of the international collaborative study. Amsterdam, Oxford, New York, Elsevier North/Holland, pp. 560-569 (Progress in Mutation Research, Volume 1).

Petzold GL & Swenberg JA (1978) Detection of DNA damage induced *in vivo* following exposure of rats to carcinogens. Cancer Res, 38: 1589-1594.

Phillips LJ & Birchard GF (1991) Regional variations in human toxic exposure in the USA: An analysis based on the national human adipose tissue survey. Arch Environ Contam Toxicol, 21: 159-168.

Phoon WH, Liang OK, & Kee CP (1975) An epidemiological study of an outbreak of jaundice in a factory. Ann Acad Med Singap, 4: 396-399.

Phoon WH, Goh KT, Lee LT, Tan KT, & Kwok SF (1983) Toxic jaundice from occupational exposure to chloroform. Med J Malays, 38: 31-34.

Plaa GL & Larson RE (1965) Relative nephrotoxicity properties of chlorinated methane, ethane and ethylene derivatives in mice. Toxicol Appl Pharmacol, 7: 34-44.

Plaa GL, Evans EA, & Hine CH (1958) Relative hepatotoxicity of seven halogenated hydrocarbons. J Pharmacol Exp Ther, 123: 224-229.

Plummer JL, Hall P de la M, Ilsley AH, Jenner MA, & Cousins MJ (1990) Influence of enzyme induction and exposure profile on liver injury due to chlorinated hydrocarbon inhalation. Pharmacol Toxicol, 67: 329-335.

Pohl LR (1979) Biochemical toxicology of chloroform. Rev Biochem Toxicol, 1: 79-107.

Pohl LR & Krishna G (1978) Deuterium isotope effect in bioactivation and hepatotoxicity of chloroform. Life Sci, 23: 1067-1072.

Pohl LR, Brooshan B, Whittaker NF, & Krishna G (1977) Phosgene: A metabolite of chloroform. Biochem Biophys Res Commun, 79: 684-691.

Pohl LR, George JW, Martin JL, & Krishna G (1979) Deuterium isotope effect in *in vivo* bioactivation of chloroform to phosgene. Biochem Pharmacol, 28: 561-563.

Pohl LR, Martin JL, & George JW (1980) Mechanism of metabolic activation of chloroform by rat liver microsomes. Biochem Pharmacol, 29: 3271-3276.

Pohl LR, Branchflower RV, Highet RJ, Martin JL, Nunn DS, Monks TJ, George JW, & Hinson JA (1981) The formation of diglutathionyl dithiocarbonate as a metabolite of chloroform, bromotrichloromethane and carbon tetrachloride. Drug Metab Dispos, 9: 334-339.

Rao KN, Virji MA, Moraca MA, Diven WF, Martin TG, & Schneider SM (1993) Role of serum markers for liver function and regeneration in the management of chloroform poisoning. J Anal Toxicol, 17: 99-102.

Ray SD & Mehendale HM (1990) Potentiation of CCl_4 and $CHCl_3$ hepatotoxicity and lethality by various alcohols. Fundam Appl Toxicol, 15: 429-440.

Reddy TV, Daniel FB, Lin EL, Stober JA, & Olson GR (1992) Chloroform inhibits the development of diethylnitrosamine-initiated, phenobarbital-promoted gamma-glutamyltranspeptidase and placental form glutathione S-transferase positive foci in rat liver. Carcinogenesis, 13: 1325-1330.

Reitz RH, Fox TR, & Quast JF (1982) Mechanistic considerations for carcinogenic risk estimation: chloroform. Environ Health Perspect, 46: 163-168.

Rem RM, Anderson ME, Daletsky SA, Misenheimer DC, & Rollius HF (1982) Chloroform materials balance (EPA Draft Report 68-02-3168).

Reuber MD (1979) Carcinogenicity of chloroform. Environ Health Perspect, 31: 171-182.

Reynolds ES & Yee AG (1967) Liver parenchymal cell injury. V. Relationships between patterns of chloromethane-C^{14} incorporation into constituents of liver *in vivo* and cellular injury. Lab Invest, 16: 591-603.

Reynolds LF & Harrison DW (1982) Studies of discharges of: benzene, chloroform and carbon tetrachloride into the aquatic environment and the best technical means for reduction of water pollution from such discharges. Brixham, Devon, ICI Brixham Laboratory (Report No. BL/A/2198).

Reynolds ES, Treinen RJ, Farrish HH, & Moslen MT (1984) Metabolism of [^{14}C] carbon tetrachloride to exhaled, excreted and bound metabolites. Biochem Pharmacol 21: 3363-3374.

Richold M & Jones M (1981) Mutagenic activity of 42 coded compounds in the Salmonella/microsome assay. In: De Serres FJ & Ashby J ed. Evaluation on short-term tests for carcinogens: Report of the international collaborative study. Amsterdam, Oxford, New York, Elsevier North/Holland, pp 314-322 (Progress in Mutation Research, Volume 1).

Robinson AB, Manly KF, Anthony MP, Catchpool JF, & Pauling L (1965) Anesthesia of Artemia larvae. Method for quantitative study. Science, 149: 1255-1258.

Roe FJC, Palmer AK, Worden AN, & Van Abbé NJ (1979) Safety evaluation of toothpaste containing chloroform. 1. Long-term studies in mice. J Environ Pathol Toxicol, 2: 799-819.

Rosenberg C, Nylund L, Aalto T, Kontsas H, Norppa H, Jäppinen P, & Vainio H (1991) Volatile organohalogen compounds from the bleaching of pulp - Occurrence and genotoxic potential in the work environment. Chemosphere, 23: 1617-1628.

Rosenkranz HS, Hyman J, & Leifer Z (1981) DNA polymerase deficient assay. In: De Serres FJ & Ashby J ed. Evaluation of short-term tests for carcinogens: Report of the international collaborative study. Amsterdam, Oxford, New York, Elsevier North/Holland, pp 210-218 (Progress in Mutation Research, Volume 1).

Rowland I & Severn B (1981) Mutagenicity of carcinogens and non-carcinogens in the Salmonella/microsome test. In: De Serres FJ & Ashby J eds. Evaluation of short-term tests for carcinogens: Report of the international collaborative study. Amsterdam, Oxford, New York, Elsevier North/Holland, pp 323-332 (Progress in Mutation Research, Volume 1).

Rubinstein D & Kanics L (1964) The conversion of carbon tetrachloride and chloroform to carbon dioxide by rat liver homogenates. Can J Biochem, 42: 1577-1585.

Ruddick JV, Villeneuve DC, & Chu I (1983) A teratological assessment of four trihalomethanes in the rat. J Environ Sci Health, B18: 333-349.

Rudolph J & Jebsen C (1983) The use of photoionization, flameionization and electron capture detectors in series for the determination of low molecular weight trace components in the non urban atmosphere. Int J Environ Anal Chem, **13**: 129-139.

Russell JW & Shadoff LA (1977) The sampling and determination of halocarbons in ambient air using concentration on porous polymer. J Chromatogr, **132**: 375-384.

Ryan DE, Koop DR, Thomas PE, Coon MJ, & Levin W (1986) Evidence that isoniazid and ethanol induce the same microsomal cytochrome P-450 in rat liver, an isozyme homologous to rabbit cytochrome P-450 isozyme 3a. Arch Biochem Biophys, **246**: 633-644.

Salamone MF, Heddle JA, & Katz M (1981) Mutagenic activity of 41 compounds in the *in vivo* micronucleus assay. In: De Serres FJ & Ashby J ed. Evaluation of short-term tests for carcinogens: Report of the international collaborative study. Amsterdam, Oxford, New York, Elsevier North/Holland, pp 686-697 (Progress in Mutation Research, Volume 1).

Salisbury S (1982) Health hazard evaluation. Charleston Laboratory (Report No. HETA-81-359-1058).

Sato A, Nakajima T, & Koyama Y (1980) Effects of chronic ethanol consumption on hepatic metabolism of aromatic and chlorinated hydrocarbons in rats. Br J Ind Med, **37**: 382-386.

Sato A, Najajiwa T, & Koyama Y (1981) Dose-related effect of a single dose of ethanol on the metabolism in rat liver of some aromatic and chlorinated hydrocarbons. Toxicol Appl Pharmacol, **60**: 8-15.

Savoure N, Maudet M, & Nicol M (1992) Toxicité du chloroforme et statut vitaminique A chez le rat. J Toxicol Clin Exp, **12**: 97-108.

Scholler KL (1966) [Electron microscope studies on rat liver cells after anaesthesia with various inhalational anaesthetics.] Anaesthesist, **15**: 145-148 (in German).

Scholler KL (1967) [The effect of halothane and chloroform on the fine structure and protein synthesis of rat's liver.] Experientia (Basel), **23**: 652-655 (in German).

Schröder HG (1965) Acute and delayed chloroform poisoning. A case report. Br J Anaesth, **37**: 971-975.

Schwetz BA, Leong BKJ, & Gehring PJ (1974) Embryo- and fetotoxicity of inhaled chloroform in rats. Toxicol Appl Pharmacol, **28**: 442-451.

Sharp DC & Parry JM (1981a) Induction of mitotic gene conversion by 41 coded compounds using the yeast culture JD1. In: De Serres FJ & Ashby J ed. Evaluation of short-term tests for carcinogens: Report of the international collaborative study. Amsterdam, Oxford, New York, Elsevier North/Holland, pp 491-501 (Progress in Mutation Research, Volume 1).

Sharp DC & Parry JM (1981b) Use of repair-deficient strains of yeast to assay the activity of 40 coded compounds. In: De Serres FJ & Ashby J ed. Evaluation of short-term tests for carcinogens: Report of the international collaborative study. Amsterdam, Oxford, New York, Elsevier North/Holland, pp 502-516 (Progress in Mutation Research, Volume 1).

Simmon VF & Shepherd GH (1981) Mutagenic activity of 42 coded compounds in the Salmonella/microsome assay. In: De Serres FJ & Ashby J ed. Evaluation of short-term tests for carcinogens: Report of the international collaborative study. Amsterdam, Oxford, New York, Elsevier North/Holland, pp 333-342 (Progress in Mutation Research, Volume 1).

Simmon VF, Kauhanen K, & Tardiff RG (1977) Mutagenic activity of chemicals identified in drinking water. In: Scott D ed. Progress in genetic toxicology. Amsterdam, Oxford, New York, Elsevier/North Holland Biomedical Press, pp 249-258.

Simpson JY (1847) On a new anaesthetic agent, more efficient than sulfuric ether. Lancet, 2: 549-550.

Sipes IG, Stripp B, Krishna G, Maling HM, & Gillette JR (1973) Enhanced hepatic microsomal activity by pretreatment of rats with acetone or isopropanol. Proc Soc Exp Biol Med, 142: 237-240.

Sipes IG, Krishna G, & Gillette JR (1977) Bioactivation of carbon tetrachloride, chloroform and bromotrichloromethane: role of cytochrome P-450. Life Sci, 20: 1541-1548.

Skopek TS, Andon BM, Kaden DA, & Thilly WG (1981) Mutagenic activity of 42 coded compounds using 8-azaguanine resistance as a genetic marker in *Salmonella typhimurium*. In: De Serres FJ & Ashby J ed. Evaluation of short-term tests for carcinogens: Report of the international collaborative study. Amsterdam, Oxford, New York, Elsevier North/Holland, pp 371-375 (Progress in Mutation Research, Volume 1).

Skrzypinska GM, Piotrowski JK, & Koralewska J (1991) The hepatotoxic action of chloroform: short-time dynamics of biochemical alterations and dose-effect relationships. Pol J Occup Med, 4(1): 77-84.

Slooff W (1979) Detection limits of a biological monitoring system based on fish respiration. Bull Environ Contam Toxicol, 23: 517-523.

Smith JH & Hook JB (1983) Mechanism of chloroform nephrotoxicity. II. *In vitro* evidence for renal metabolism of chloroform in mice. Toxicol Appl Pharmacol, 70: 480-485.

Smith JH & Hook JB (1984) Mechanism of chloroform nephrotoxicity. III. Renal and hepatic microsomal metabolism of chloroform in mice. Toxicol Appl Pharmacol, 73: 511-524.

Smith AA, Volpitto PP, Gramling ZW, DeVore MB, & Glassman AB (1973) Chloroform, haloethane and regional anesthesia: A comparative study. Anesth Analg, 52: 1-11.

Smith JH, Maita K, Sleight SD, & Hook JB (1983) Mechanism of nephrotoxicity. I. Time course of chloroform toxicity in male and female mice. Toxicol Appl Pharmacol, 70: 467-479.

Smith JH, Maita K, Sleight SD, & Hook JB (1984) Effect of sex hormones status on chloroform nephrotoxicity and renal mixed function oxidase in mice. Toxicology, 30: 305-316.

Smith JH, Hewitt WR, & Hook JB (1985) Role of intrarenal biotransformation in chloroform-induced nephrotoxicity in rats. Toxicol Appl Pharmacol, 79: 166-174.

Spence JW, Philip LH, Hanst PL, & Gray BW (1976) Atmospheric oxidation of methyl chloride, methylene chloride and chloroform. J Air Pollut Control Assoc, 26: 994.

Stacey NH (1987) Assessment of the toxicity of chemical mixtures with isolated rat hepatocytes: cadmium and chloroform. Fundam Appl Toxicol, 9: 616-622.

Stander GJ (1980) Micro-organic compounds in the water environment and their impact on the quality of potable water supplies. Water S Afr, 6: 1-14.

Stevens JL & Anders MW (1981a) Effect of cysteine, diethylmaleate and phenobarbital treatments on the hepatotoxicity of [^{1}H]- and [^{2}H]-chloroform. Chem-Biol Interact, 37: 207-217.

Stevens JL & Anders MW (1981b) Metabolism of haloforms to carbon monoxide. IV. Studies on the reaction mechanism *in vivo*. Chem-Biol Interact, 37: 365-374.

Stewart ME, Blogoslawski WJ, Hsu RY, & Helz GR (1979) By-products of oxidative biocides: toxicity to oyster larvae. Mar Pollut Bull, 10: 166-169.

Storms WW (1973) Chloroform parties. J Am Med Assoc, 255: 160.

Strand SE & Shippert L (1986) Oxidation of chloroform in an aerobic soil exposed to natural gas. Appl Environ Microbiol, 52: 203-205.

Sturrock J (1977) Lack of mutagenic effect of halothane or chloroform on cultured cells using the azaguanine test system. Br J Anaesth, 49: 207-210.

Styles JA (1979) Cell transformation assays. In: Paget GE ed. Topics in toxicology - Mutagens in sub-mammalian systems: Status and significance. Baltimore, Maryland, University Park Press, pp 147-161.

Styles JA (1981) Activity of 42 coded compounds in the BHK-21 cell transformation test. In: De Serres FJ & Ashby J ed. Evaluation of short-term tests for carcinogens: Report of the international collaborative study. Amsterdam, Oxford, New York, Elsevier North/Holland, pp 638-646 (Progress in Mutation Research, Volume 1).

Su C & Goldberg E (1976) Environmental concentration and fluxes of some halocarbons. Mar Pollut Transf, 353-373.

Taketomo AP & Grimsrud E (1977) An analysis of halocarbons in the air of several working and living environments. Proc Mont Acad Sci, 37: 128-134.

Taylor DC, Brown DM, Keeble R, & Langley PF (1974) Metabolism of chloroform. II. A sex difference in the metabolism of (^{14}C) chloroform in mice. Xenobiotica, 4: 165-174.

Taylor GJ, Drew RT, Lores EM, & Clemmer TA (1976) Cardiac depression by haloalkane propellants, solvents and inhalation anaesthetics in rabbits. Toxicol Appl Pharmacol, 38: 379-387.

Temmerman IFMM & Quaghebeur DJM (1990) Analysis of trihalomethanes by direct aqueous injection (THM-DAI). Short communications. J High Res Chromatogr, 13: 379-381.

Testai E & Vittozzi L (1986) Biochemical alterations elicited in rat liver microsomes by oxidation and reduction products of chloroform metabolism. Chem-Biol Interact, **59**: 157-171.

Testai E, Di Marzio S, & Vittozzi L (1990) Multiple activation of chloroform in hepatic microsomes from uninduced B6C3F1 mice. Toxicol Appl Pharmacol, **104**: 496-503.

Testai, E, Keizer J, Pacifici GM, & Vittozzi L (1991) Chloroform bioactivation by microsomes from colonic and ileal mucosa of rat and man. Toxicol Lett, **57**: 19-27.

Thompson DJ, Warner SD, & Robinson VB (1974) Teratology studies on orally administered chloroform in the rat and rabbit. Toxicol Appl Pharmacol, **29**: 348-357.

Thomson JA (1981) Mutagenic activity of 42 coded compounds in the Lambda induction assay. In: De Serres FJ & Ashby J ed. Evaluation of short-term tests for carcinogens: Report of the international collaborative study. Amsterdam, Oxford, New York, Elsevier North/Holland, pp 224-235 (Progress in Mutation Research, Volume 1).

Timms RM & Moser KM (1975) Toxicity secondary to intravenously administered chloroform in humans. Arch Intern Med, **135**: 1601-1603.

Tomasi A, Albano E, Biasi F, Slater TF, Vannini V, & Dianzani MU (1985) Activation of chloroform and related trihalomethanes to free radical intermediates in isolated hepatocytes and in the rat *in vivo* as detected by the ESR-spin trapping technique. Chem-Biol Interact, **55**: 303-316.

Topham JC (1980) Do induced sperm-head abnormalities in mice specifically identify mammalian mutagens rather than carcinogens? Mutat Res, **74**: 379-387.

Topham JC (1981) Evaluation of some chemicals by the sperm morphology assay. In: De Serres FJ & Ashby J ed. Evaluation of short-term tests for carcinogens: Report of the international collaborative study. Amsterdam, Oxford, New York, Elsevier North/Holland, pp 718-720 (Progress in Mutation Research, Volume 1).

Torkelson TR, Oyen F, & Rowe VK (1976) The toxicity of chloroform as determined by single and repeated exposure of laboratory animals. Am Ind Hyg Assoc J, **37**: 697-705.

Toxicology and Environmental Health Institute of Munich Technical University (1992) [Recommendations on chloroform/emission data. BUA plenary session in Merseburg, 24-25 August 1992.] Berlin, Federal Office of the Environment (BUA) (in German).

Trueman RW (1981) Activity of 42 coded compounds in the Salmonella reverse mutation test. In: De Serres FJ & Ashby J ed. Evaluation of short-term tests for carcinogens: Report of the international collaborative study. Amsterdam, Oxford, New York, Elsevier North/Holland, pp 343-350 (Progress in Mutation Research, Volume 1).

Tsuchimoto T & Matter BE (1981) Activity of coded compounds in the micronucleus test. In: De Serres FJ & Ashby J ed. Evaluation of short-term tests for carcinogens: Report of the international collaborative study. Amsterdam, Oxford, New York, Elsevier North/Holland, pp 705-711 (Progress in Mutation Research, Volume 1).

Tsuruta H (1975) Percutaneous absorption of organic solvents. Ind Health, **13**: 227-236.

Tumasonis CF, McMartin DN, & Bush B (1985) Lifetime toxicity of chloroform and bromodichloromethane when administered over a lifetime in rats. Ecotoxicol Environ Saf, 9: 233-240.

Tweats DJ (1981) Activity of 42 coded compounds in a differential killing test using *Escherichia coli* strains WP2, WP67 (uvra pol A), and CM871 (uvrA AlexA recA). In: De Serres FJ & Ashby J ed. Evaluation of short-term tests for carcinogens: Report of the international collaborative study. Amsterdam, Oxford, New York, Elsevier North/Holland, pp 199-209 (Progress in Mutation Research, Volume 1).

Tyson CA, Hawk-Prather K, Story DL, & Gould DH (1983) Correlations of *in vitro* and *in vivo* hepatotoxicity for five haloalkanes. Toxicol Appl Pharmacol, 70: 289-302.

Uchrin CG & Mangels G (1986) Chloroform sorption to New Jersey coastal plain ground water aquifer solids. Environ Toxicol Chem, 5: 339-343.

Uehleke H & Werner T (1975) A comparative study on the irreversible binding of labelled halothane, trichlorofluoromethane, chloroform and carbon tetrachloride to hepatic protein and lipids *in vitro* and *in vivo*. Arch Toxicol, 34: 289-308.

Uehleke H, Greim H, Krämer M, & Werner (1976) Covalent binding of haloalkanes to liver constituents but absence of mutagenicity on bacteria in metabolising test system. Mutat Res, 38: 114.

Uehleke H, Werner T, Greim H, & Krämer M (1977) Metabolic activation of haloethanes and tests *in vitro* for mutagenicity. Xenobiotica, 7: 393-400.

Ullrich D (1982) [Organic halogen compounds in the air of some Berlin indoor swimming pools.] WoBoLu-Berlin, 1: 50-52 (in German).

US EPA (1971) Compendium of registered pesticides. Washington, DC, US Environmental Protection Agency, p III-C-19.

US EPA (1984) Locating and estimating air emissions from sources of chloroform. US Washington, DC, Environmental Protection Agency (Report PB-84-200617).

US EPA (1992) Technical Support Division (TSD). Disinfection by-products field study data base. Washington, DC, US Environmental Protection Agency, Office of Ground Water and Drinking Water, Technical Support Division.

US FDA (US Food and Drug Administration (1976) Chloroform as an ingredient of human drug and cosmetic products. Fed Reg, 41: 26842-26845.

US NIOSH (1984) Manual of analytical methods - Volume 1: Method 1003. Cincinnati, Ohio, National Institute for Occupational Safety and Health.

US NIOSH (1989) National occupational exposure survey (NOES) as of March 29, 1989. Cincinnati, Ohio, National Institute for Occupational Safety and Health.

Van Abbé NJ, Green TJ, Jones E, Richold M, & Roe FJC (1982) Bacterial mutagenicity studies on chloroform *in vitro*. Food Cosmet Toxicol, 20: 557-561.

Van Beelen P & Van Keulen F (1990) The kinetics of the degradation of chloroform and benzene in anaerobic sediment from the river Rhine. Hydrobiol Bull, 24: 13-21.

Van der Heijden CA, Speijers GJA, Ros JPM, Huldy HJ, Besemer AC, Lanting RW, Maas RJM, Heijna-Merkus E, Bergshoeff G, Gerlofsma A, Mennes WC, Van der Most PFJ, De Vrijer FL, Janssen PCJM, Knaap AGAC, Huijgen C, Duiser JA, & De Jong P (1986) Criteria document on chloroform. Bilthoven The Netherlands, National Institute of Public Health and Environmental Protection (Report No. 738513004).

Van Dyke RA, Chenoweth MB, & Van Poznak A (1964) Metabolism of volatile anaesthetics-I. Conversion *in vivo* of several anaesthetics to $^{14}CO_2$ and chloride. Biochem Pharmacol, 13: 1239-1247.

Van Luin AB & Van Starkenburg W (1984) Hazardous substances in waste water. Water Sci Tech, 17: 843-853.

Van Tassel S, Amalfitano N, & Narang RS (1981) Determination of arenes and volatile halo-organic compounds in air at microgram per cubic meter levels by gas chromatography. Anal Chem, 53: 2130-2135.

Veith GD, Macek KJ, Petrocelli SR, & Carroll J (1978) An evaluation of using partition coefficients and water solubility to estimate bioconcentration factors for organic chemicals in fish. In: Eaton JG, Parrish PR, & Hendricks AC ed. Aquatic toxicology. Proceedings of the Third Annual Symposium on Aquatic Toxicology. Philadelphia, Pennsylvania, American Society for Testing and Materials, pp 116-129 (STP 707).

Venitt S & Crofton-Sleigh C (1981) Mutagenicity of 42 coded compounds in a bacterial assay using *Escherichia coli* and *Salmonella typhimurium*. In: De Serres FJ & Ashby J ed. Evaluation of short-term tests for carcinogens: Report of the international collaborative study. Amsterdam, Oxford, New York, Elsevier North/Holland, pp 351-360 (Progress in Mutation Research, Volume 1).

Verschueren U (1983) Handbook of environmental data on organic chemicals, 2nd ed. New York, Van Nostrand Reinhold Company, pp 367-369.

Vézina M, Kobusch AB, Du Souich P, Greselin E, & Plaa GL (1990) Potentiation of chloroform-induced hepatotoxicity by methyl isobutyl ketone and two metabolites. Can J Physiol Pharmacol, 68: 1055-1061.

Vittozzi L, Testai E, & De Biasi A (1991) Multiple bioactivation of chloroform: a comparison between man and experimental animals. Adv Exp Med Biol, 283: 665-667.

Vogel E, Blijleven WGH, Kortselius MJH, & Zijlstra JA (1981) Mutagenic activity of 17 coded compounds in the sex-linked recessive lethal test in *Drosophila melanogaster*. In: De Serres FJ & Ashby J ed. Evaluation of short-term tests for carcinogens: Report of the international collaborative study. Amsterdam, Oxford, New York, Elsevier North/Holland, pp 660-665 (Progress in Mutation Research, Volume 1).

Von Oettingen WF (1964) The halogenated hydrocarbons of industrial and toxicological importance. Amsterdam, Oxford, New York, Elsevier Science Publishers, pp 77-108.

Von Oettingen WF, Powell CC, Sharpless NE, Alford WC, & Pecoza LJ (1950) Comparative studies of the toxicity and pharmacodynamic action of chlorinated methanes with special reference to their physical and chemical action. Arch Int Pharmacodyn, 81: 17-34.

Wallace LA (1987) The total exposure assessment methodology (TEAM) study: Summary and analysis. Volume I (EPA/600/6 - 87/002a).

Wallace LA, Pellizzari E, Hartwell T, Rosenzweig M, Erickson M, Sparacino, C & Zelon H (1984) Personal exposure to volatile organic compounds. I. Direct measurements in breathing-zone air, drinking water, food and exhaled breath. Environ Res, 35: 293-319.

Wecher RA & Scher S (1982) Bioassay procedures for identifying genotoxic agents using light emitting bacteria as indicator organisms. In: Seno M & Pazzagli M ed. Luminescent assays: perspectives in endocrinology and clinical chemistry. New York, Raven Press Ltd, pp 109-113.

Westrick JJ, Mello JW, & Thomas RF (1989) The groundwater supply survey. J Am Water Works Assoc, 76: 52-59.

White AE, Takehisa S, Eger EI, Wolff S, & Stevens WC (1979) Sister chromatid exchanges induced by inhaled anaesthetics. Anesthesiology, 50: 426-430.

WHO (1993) Guidelines for drinking-water quality, 2nd ed. Volume 1: Recommendations. Geneva, World Health Organization.

WHO (in press) IPCS Environmental Health Criteria 170: Assessing human health risks of chemicals: Derivation of guidance values for health-based exposure limits. Geneva, World Health Organization.

Williams DT, Olson R, Bothwell PD, Murphy KI, & Robertson JL (1980) Trihalomethane levels in Canadian drinking water. Environ Sci Res, 16: 503-512.

Wilson JT, Enfield CG, Dunlap WJ, Cosby RL, Foster DA, & Baskin LB (1981) Transport and fate of selected organic pollutants in a sandy soil. J Environ Qual, 10: 501-506.

Windholz M ed. (1983) The Merck index: an encyclopedia of chemicals, drugs, and biologicals, 10th ed. Rahway, New Jersey, Merck & Co., Inc.

Winslow SG & Gerstner HB (1978) Health aspects of chloroform. A review. Drug Chem Toxicol, 1: 259-275.

Withey JR & Collins BT (1980) Chlorinated aliphatic hydrocarbons used in the foods industry: the comparative pharmacokinetics of methylene chloride, 1,2-dichloroethane, chloroform and trichloroethylene after i.v. administration in the rat. J Environ Pathol Toxicol, 3: 313-332.

Withey JR & Karpinski K (1985) The fetal distribution of some aliphatic chlorinated hydrocarbons in the rat after vapour phase exposure. Biol Res Pregnancy, 6: 79-88.

Withey JR, Collins BT, & Collins PG (1983) Effect of vehicle on the pharmacokinetics and uptake of four halogenated hydrocarbons by the gastrointestinal tract of the rat. J Appl Toxicol, 3: 249-253.

Wolf CR, Mansuy D, Nastainczyk W, Deutschmann G, & Ullrich V (1977) The reduction of polyhalogenated methanes by liver microsomal cytochrome P-450. Mol Pharmacol, 13: 698-705.

Youssefi M, Faust SD, & Zenchelsky ST (1978) Rapid determination of light halogenated hydrocarbons in urine. Clin Chem, **24**: 1109-1111.

Zaleska-Rutczynska Z & Krus S (1973) Genetic aspects of the high and low sensitivity to chloroform of male mice of various inbred strains and their crosses. Pol Med Sci Hist Bull Abstr, **1**: 245-250.

Zimmermann FK & Scheel I (1981) Induction of mitotic gene conversion in strain D7 of *Saccharomyces cerevisiae* by 42 coded chemicals. In: De Serres FJ & Ashby J ed. Evaluation of short-term tests for carcinogens: Report of the international collaborative study. Amsterdam, Oxford, New York, Elsevier North/Holland, pp 481-490 (Progress in Mutation Research, Volume 1).

Zoeteman BCJ, Hrubec J, de Greef E, & Kool HJ (1982) Mutagenic activity associated with by-products of drinking water disinfection by chlorine, chlorine dioxide, ozone and UV-irradiation. Environ Health Perspect, **46**: 197-205.

RESUME

Le chloroforme se présente sous la forme d'un liquide volatil, limpide et incolore, à l'odeur caractéristique et au goût âcre et douceâtre. Il peut être décomposé par voie photochimique, il n'est pas inflammable et il est soluble dans la plupart des solvants organiques. Toutefois sa solubilité dans l'eau est limitée. Lors de la décomposition chimique, il peut y avoir formation de phosgène et d'acide chlorhydrique.

Le chloroforme s'emploie dans certaines formulations de pesticides, comme solvant et comme intermédiaire dans la fabrication de certains dérivés. Son utilisation comme anesthésique ou dans des spécialités pharmaceutiques est interdite dans un certain nombre de pays. La production de chloroforme à des fins commerciales a atteint 440 000 tonnes en 1987. Du chloroforme se forme également en quantités appréciables lors de la chloration de l'eau et du blanchiment de la pâte à papier.

L'analyse de l'air, de l'eau et d'échantillons biologiques pour la recherche et le dosage du chloroforme peut s'effectuer selon plusieurs méthodes. La majorité d'entre elles consiste en une injection directe sur colonne, une adsorption sur un adsorbant activé ou une condensation dans un piège froid; on procède ensuite à une désorption ou à une extraction par un solvant qui est ensuite chassé avant analyse finale par chromatographie en phase gazeuse.

On pense que la majeure partie du chloroforme présent dans l'eau finit par passer dans l'air, en raison de la volatilité de ce composé. Le temps de séjour du chloroforme dans l'atmosphère est de plusieurs mois et il en est éliminé après transformation chimique. Il résiste à la biodégradation aérobie par les bactéries du sol et des nappes phréatiques qui se développent sur des substrats endogènes ou en présence d'un supplément d'acétate. Il peut y avoir biodégradation en anaérobiose. La bioconcentration est faible chez les poissons d'eau douce. La dépuration est rapide.

D'après l'estimation de l'exposition moyenne due aux divers milieux, on pense que la population générale est principalement exposée au chloroforme par l'intermédiaire de la nourriture, de l'eau de boisson et de l'air intérieur, dans des proportions à peu près égales. L'absorption estimative à partir de l'air intérieur est cependant beaucoup moindre. L'absorption moyenne totale estimative est d'environ 2 μg/kg de poids corporel, par jour. Les données disponibles indiquent également que l'utilisation domestique de l'eau contribue de façon très importante à la concentration du chloroforme dans l'air intérieur et par voie de conséquence à l'exposition totale. Pour certaines personnes qui vivent dans des habitations où l'eau de distribution renferme des concentrations relativement élevées de chloroforme, on estime que l'absorption totale peut aller jusqu'à 10 μg/kg de poids corporel et par jour.

Une fois administré par voie orale, le chloroforme est bien résorbé chez l'animal et l'homme, mais la cinétique d'absorption dépend du véhicule. Chez l'homme, après exposition par la voie respiratoire, 60 à 80% de la dose inhalée sont absorbés. Les principaux facteurs qui agissent sur la cinétique d'absorption du chloroforme après inhalation sont la concentration ainsi que la capacité de métabolisation, qui dépend de l'espèce. Chez l'homme et l'animal, le chloroforme est rapidement résorbé par la peau et l'on a montré qu'il pouvait être également absorbé par voie percutanée dans une proportion importante à partir de l'eau lors d'une douche. Il semble que l'hydratation de l'épiderme accélère la résorption du chloroforme.

Le chloroforme se répartit dans l'ensemble de l'organisme. C'est dans les graisses, le sang, le foie, les reins, les poumons et le système nerveux que l'on trouve les plus fortes concentrations tissulaires. La répartition du chloroforme dépend de la voie d'exposition; la dose est plus forte dans les tissus extra-hépatiques après inhalation ou absorption percutanée qu'après ingestion. On a montré que chez plusieurs espèces animales et chez l'homme, le chloroforme pouvait traverser la barrière placentaire. Il s'élimine essentiellement dans l'air expiré sous forme de dioxyde de carbone. Non métabolisé, il demeure plus longtemps dans les graisses que dans les autres tissus.

La biotransformation oxydative du chloroforme en trichlorométhanol est catalysée par le cytochrome P-450. Le trichlorométhanol produit, par élimination d'HCl, un intermédiaire réactif, le phosgène. Le phosgène peut être détoxifié en dioxyde de carbone par réaction avec l'eau ou en divers adduits par réaction avec des thiols, notamment le glutathion ou la cystéine. La réaction du phosgène sur les protéines tissulaires entraîne des lésions cellulaires et la mort. La liaison des métabolites du chloroforme à l'ADN est limitée. Le chloroforme peut également subir une biotransformation réductrice catalysée par le P-450, qui donne naissance au radical dichlorométhyl, lequel se fixe ensuite par liaison covalente aux lipides tissulaires. On n'a pas déterminé si cette biotransformation réductrice jouait également un rôle dans la cytotoxicité du chloroforme.

Chez l'animal et l'homme exposés à du chloroforme, le chloroforme est éliminé d'une part sous forme de dioxyde de carbone et d'autre part sous forme inchangée. La fraction de la dose qui est éliminée sous forme de dioxyde de carbone varie avec cette dose et l'espèce en cause. La vitesse de biotransformation en dioxyde de carbone est plus élevée dans les microsomes hépatiques et rénaux des rongeurs (hamster, souris, rat) que dans ceux de l'homme. La biotransformation du chloroforme est également plus rapide dans les microsomes rénaux des souris que dans ceux des rats.

En ce qui concerne la toxicité aiguë, c'est le foie qui est l'organe-cible chez le rat et plusieurs souches de souris. Les lésions hépatiques se caractérisent essentiellement, au début, par une infiltration graisseuse et une ballonisation des cellules, qui évoluent vers une nécrose centrilobulaire, puis une nécrose massive. Le rein est l'organe-cible chez les souris mâles appartenant à des souches plus sensibles. Au niveau du rein, les lésions débutent par une dégénérescence hydropigène qui évolue vers la nécrose des tubules proximaux. On n'a pas observé de toxicité rénale importante chez les femelles d'aucune souche de souris.

La toxicité aiguë varie en fonction de la souche, du sexe et du véhicule. Chez la souris, la DL_{50} par voie orale varie de 36 à 1366 mg/kg de poids corporel alors que chez le rat, elle peut aller de 450 à 2000 mg de chloroforme par kg de poids corporel. Après une seule exposition de 4 heures par voie respiratoire, on a observé des effets toxiques sur le foie chez la souris et le rat à des concentrations de chloroforme respectivement égales à 490 et 1410 mg/m^3.

Ce sont les lésions du foie qui sont l'effet toxique du chloroforme le plus universellement observé. La gravité de ces effets par dose unitaire administrée dépend de l'espèce, du véhicule et du mode d'administration du chloroforme. La dose la plus faible à laquelle on ait observé ces lésions est de 15 mg/kg de poids corporel et par jour, administrée à des chiens "beagle" dans une base de pâte dentifrice, pendant une période de 7,5 années. On n'a pas recherché s'il y avait des effets à des doses plus faibles.

Chez les autres espèces, les doses nécessaires pour produire des effets hépatotoxiques sont un peu plus élevées. Bien qu'au cours de ces différentes études, la durée d'exposition ait été variable, on a pu fixer la concentration sans effets nocifs observables à 15-125 mg/kg de poids corporel et par jour.

Les effets au niveau du rein ont été observés chez des mâles appartenant à des souches sensibles de souris ainsi que chez des rats F-344. Ces effets étaient graves chez les mâles appartenant à une souche de souris particulièrement sensible, à des doses ne dépassant pas 36 mg/kg de poids corporel et par jour.

Chez des rats F-344 à qui l'on avait fait inhaler du chloroforme 7 jours de suite, tous les jours pendant 6 heures, on a observé une atrophie des glandes de Bowman ainsi que la présence d'os néoformés dans les cornets du nez. La dose sans effets observables correspondante se situait à 14,7 mg/m^3 (3 ppm). Des études à long terme se poursuivent afin d'évaluer la portée de ces effets.

On a constaté l'apparition de tumeurs hépatiques chez des souris à qui l'on avait administré par gavage des doses quotidiennes de chloroforme dans de l'huile de maïs, à raison de 138 à 477 mg/kg de poids corporel. Toutefois, lorsque des doses analogues étaient administrées dans l'eau de boisson, le chloroforme était sans influence sur la proportion des tumeurs hépatiques qui se formaient chez ces souris. De plus, lors d'études sur le caractère promoteur éventuel de ce composé, on a observé, qu'administré dans l'eau de boisson, le chloroforme avait en fait une action inhibitrice sur la formation de tumeurs du foie provoquées chez la souris avec de la diéthylnitrosamine comme initiateur. Le véhicule utilisé ou la manière d'administrer le chloroforme conditionne donc de façon importante son pouvoir tumoro-inducteur au niveau du foie chez la souris.

Le chloroforme a produit des tumeurs rénales chez des rats qui en avaient reçu quotidiennement par gavage, dans de l'huile de maïs, des doses allant de 90 à 200 mg/kg de poids corporel. Toutefois, chez cette espèce, les résultats se sont révélés analogues lorsque le produit était administré dans l'eau de boisson, ce qui indique que les effets ne dépendent pas entièrement du véhicule utilisé.

Il semble que les effets cancérogènes du chloroforme sur le foie et le rein des rongeurs soient étroitement liés à son action cytotoxique ainsi qu'aux effets que ce composé exerce sur la réplication cellulaire dans les organes-cibles. On a constaté que ces derniers effets suivaient de près les modifications de la réponse cancérogène au chloroforme en fonction du type de véhicule et du mode d'administration. A la lumière des données disponibles, il semble que le chloroforme ne soit guère capable d'induire des mutations géniques ou d'autres types de lésions directes de l'ADN. En outre, le chloroforme ne semble pas non plus capable de jouer le rôle d'initiateur tumoral au niveau du foie chez la souris ni d'induire une synthèse non programmée de l'ADN *in vivo*. En revanche, lorsqu'il est administré dans un véhicule huileux, le chloroforme peut se révéler un promoteur efficace des tumeurs hépatiques. Par conséquent, il est probable que, lors de l'administration prolongée de chloroforme, la cytotoxicité de ce composé et la prolifération cellulaire qu'il détermine sont les causes les plus importantes de la formation de tumeurs hépatiques et rénales chez les rongeurs.

On dispose de quelques données limitées selon lesquelles le chloroforme serait toxique pour le foetus, mais uniquement à des doses auxquelles il est également toxique pour la mère.

En général, le chloroforme détermine les mêmes symptômes toxiques chez l'homme que chez l'animal. Chez l'homme, l'anesthésie peut entraîner la mort par suite d'arythmie et d'insuffisance respiratoire et cardiaque. On a également observé chez l'homme une nécrose des tubules rénaux et une insuffisance rénale. Les doses les plus faibles pour lesquelles des cas de toxicité hépatique due à une exposition professionnelle au chloroforme ont fait l'objet de rapports, se situaient dans les limites de 80 à 160 mg/m^3 (durée d'exposition de moins de 4 mois) selon une étude et allaient de 10 à 1000 mg/m^3 (durée d'exposition: 1 à 4 ans) selon une autre étude. On estime que la dose mortelle moyenne par voie orale pour un adulte est d'environ 45 g, mais on note d'importantes différences de sensibilité selon les individus. On est fondé à croire, selon certaines études épidémiologiques, qu'il existe une association entre l'exposition aux sous-produits des désinfectants présents dans l'eau de boisson et les cancers colorectaux ou vésicaux. Cependant, ces études souffrent de la présence de facteurs de confusion, entre autres faiblesses. Les preuves avancées à l'appui de la cancérogénicité pour l'homme de l'eau de boisson chlorée, sont insuffisantes. En outre, la présence de sous-produits des désinfectants utilisés ne peut être attribuée au chloroforme lui-même.

Le chloroforme est toxique pour les stages embryo-larvaires de certaines espèces d'amphibiens et de poissons. La CL_{50} la plus faible dont il ait été fait état, se situait à 0,3 mg/litre pour les stades embryo-larvaires de *Hyla crucifer*. Le chloroforme est moins toxique pour les poissons et pour la daphnie *Daphnia magna*. Pour plusieurs espèces de poissons, les valeurs de la CL_{50} se situent dans les limites de 18 à 191 mg/litre. Il n'y a guère de différences de sensibilité entre les poissons d'eau douce et les poissons de mer. En ce qui concerne *Daphnia magna*, la valeur la plus faible de la CL_{50} qui ait été signalée, était de 29 mg/litre. Le chloroforme est peu toxique pour les algues et autres microorganismes.

Le Groupe de travail a estimé que les données disponibles étaient suffisantes pour établir une dose journalière tolérable (DJT) pour les effets non cancérogènes du chloroforme, ainsi qu'une dose spécifiquement liée au risque d'effets cancérogènes, sur la base des études effectuées chez l'animal; les valeurs ainsi fixées serviront de guide pour l'établissement de limites d'exposition par les autorités compétentes. Cependant, il est rappelé que lorsque les conditions locales imposent un choix entre le respect des limites microbiologiques ou celles qui concernent la présence de sous-produits de désinfection tels que le chloroforme, c'est la qualité microbiologique qui doit toujours l'emporter. Il ne faut *jamais* transiger sur l'efficacité de la désinfection.

En se fondant sur l'étude de Heywood et al. (1979) et en introduisant un facteur d'incertitude de 1000 (x10 pour les variations interspécifiques, x10 pour les variations intraspécifiques et x10 pour l'utilisation d'une dose avec effet plutôt que d'une dose sans effet lors d'une étude subchronique), on obtient une DJT de 15 µg/kg de poids corporel; il faut rappeler que cette étude avait révélé l'existence d'une légère hépatotoxicité (à savoir une augmentation des enzymes hépatiques sériques et des kystes graisseux) chez des chiens "beagle" à qui l'on avait fait ingérer pendant 7,5 ans, une pâte dentifrice contenant du chloroforme à la dose de 15 mg/kg de poids corporel et par jour.

En se fondant sur ce que l'on sait du mécanisme de ces phénomènes, la méthode que l'on juge la mieux adaptée pour obtenir une valeur-guide consiste à diviser la valeur de la concentration sans effet observable sur la prolifération cellulaire par un certain facteur d'incertitude. C'est ainsi que si l'on utilise la valeur de la dose sans effets observables obtenue par Larson et al. (1993b) pour la cytoléthalité et la prolifération cellulaire chez des souris B6C3F$_1$ qui avaient reçu pendant 3 semaines, dans de l'huile de maïs, une dose quotidienne de chloroforme équivalant à 10 mg/kg de poids corporel, et en introduisant un facteur d'incertitude de 1000 (x10 pour les variations interspécifiques, x10 pour les variations intraspécifiques et x10 pour la gravité de l'effet, c'est-à-dire la cancérogénicité et parce qu'il s'agit d'une étude subchronique), on obtient une DJT de 10 μg/kg de poids corporel.

On admet que les tumeurs rénales observées chez le rat peuvent également être liées à l'action létale du chloroforme sur les cellules et à ses effets sur leur prolifération. Cependant, étant donné que l'on ne possède pas de données sur la prolifération cellulaire chez les souches où l'on a observé des tumeurs et qu'en outre, ce que l'on peut savoir de cet effet et de l'effet létal du chloroforme sur les cellules n'a été observé qu'à court terme (un seul gavage et une exposition par voie respiratoire de 7 jours), on estime qu'il est prématuré de s'écarter du modèle par défaut (c'est-à-dire multistade linéarisé) pour l'estimation du risque de cancer sur la durée de vie. D'après l'étude de Jorgenson et al. (1985) qui portait sur l'induction de tumeurs rénales (adénomes et adénocarcinomes), on a fixé à 8,2 μg/kg de poids corporel et par jour, la dose quotidienne totale jugée capable de produire un excès de risque de 10^{-5} sur toute la durée de la vie.

La concentration de chloroforme dans les eaux de surface est généralement faible et ne semble pas présenter de danger pour les organismes aquatiques. Toutefois, la décharge ou le déversement de produits industriels pourrait entraîner la présence de concentrations plus élevées de chloroforme dans ces eaux et les rendre dangereuses pour les stades embryo-larvaires de certaines espèces aquatiques.

RESUMEN

El cloroformo es un líquido transparente, incoloro y volátil, con un olor característico y un sabor dulce ardiente. Se degrada fotoquímicamente, no es inflamable y es soluble en la mayor parte de los disolventes orgánicos. Sin embargo, su solubilidad en agua es limitada. Por degradación química del mismo pueden formarse fosgeno y ácido hidroclorhídrico.

El cloroformo se utiliza en la formulación de plaguicidas, como disolvente y como intermedio químico. Su utilización como anestésico y en especialidades farmacéuticas está prohibida en algunos países. La producción comercial ascendió a 440 000 toneladas en 1987. También se producen cantidades apreciables de cloroformo en la cloración del agua y en el blanqueado de la pasta papelera.

Existen varios métodos analíticos para determinar la presencia de cloroformo en el aire, el agua y los materiales biológicos. La mayor parte de esos métodos se basan en la inyección directa en columna, la adsorción en adsorbentes activados o la condensación en una cámara fría y posteriormente la desorción o evaporación mediante la extracción por disolventes o el calentamiento y el subsiguiente análisis por cromatografía de gases.

Se supone que la mayor parte del cloroformo presente en el agua se transfiere finalmente al aire debido a su volatilidad. El cloroformo tiene un tiempo de residencia en la atmósfera de varios meses y desaparece de la misma por transformación química. Es resistente a la biodegradación por la población microbiana aeróbica de los suelos y de las capas acuíferas que viven en substratos endógenos o con el suplemento de acetato. La biodegradación es posible en condiciones anaeróbicas. La bioconcentración en los peces de agua dulce es baja. La depuración es rápida.

Las estimaciones de la exposición media calculadas a partir de diversos medios indican que la población en general está expuesta al cloroformo principalmente a través de los alimentos, el agua de bebida y el aire de los interiores en cantidades aproximadamente equivalentes. La inhalación estimada por conducto del aire exterior es considerablemente menor. La ingesta media estimada total es de aproximadamente 2 μg/kg de peso corporal por día. Los datos disponibles también indican que el agua de uso doméstico contribuye considerablemente a los niveles de cloroformo en el aire de los interiores y a la exposición total. La ingesta total estimada de algunos individuos que viven en lugares con un abastecimiento de agua corriente con concentraciones relativamente elevadas de cloroformo asciende a 10 μg/kg de peso corporal por día.

Los animales y los seres humanos absorben bien el cloroformo después de la administración por vía oral, pero la cinética de la absorción depende del vehículo suministrado. Tras la exposición por inhalación, los seres humanos absorben del 60 al 80% de la cantidad inhalada. Los factores principales que afectan a la cinética de la absorción del cloroformo después de la inhalación son su concentración y la capacidad metabólica específica de la especie. Los seres humanos y los animales lo absorben fácilmente a través de la piel y se ha demostrado que durante la ducha la absorción dérmica del cloroformo del agua es apreciable. La hidratación de la piel parece acelerar la absorción de cloroformo.

El cloroformo se distribuye en todo el cuerpo. Los niveles tisulares más elevados se alcanzan en el tejido adiposo, la sangre, el hígado, los riñones, los pulmones y el sistema nervioso. La distribución depende de la vía de exposición; los tejidos extrahepáticos reciben una dosis más elevada del cloroformo inhalado o absorbido por la piel que del cloroformo ingerido. Se ha demostrado que en varias especies animales y en el ser humano el cloroformo se transfiere a través de la placenta. El cloroformo se elimina principalmente como dióxido de carbono exhalado. El cloroformo no metabolizado se mantiene más tiempo en el tejido adiposo que en cualquier otro tejido.

El citocromo P-450 cataliza la biotransformación oxidativa del cloroformo en triclorometanol. La pérdida de HCl del triclorometanol produce fosgeno como reactivo intermedio. El fosgeno puede destoxificarse por reacción con el agua produciendo dióxido de carbono o con tioles, inclusive con glutatión o cisteína, produciendo aductos. La reacción del fosgeno con proteínas tisulares está asociada con daño y necrosis celulares. Se observa un escaso enlace de los metabolitos del cloroformo con el ADN. El cloroformo también es objeto de una biotransformación reductiva catalizada por el P-450 que produce radicales de diclorometilo y éstos contraen enlaces covalentes con los lípidos tisulares. No se ha determinado el papel de la biotransformación reductiva en la citotoxicidad del cloroformo.

Los animales y los seres humanos expuestos al cloroformo eliminan con el aire espirado el dióxido de carbono y el cloroformo que no se ha transformado. La fracción de dosis eliminada como dióxido de carbono varía según la dosis y la especie. La tasa de biotransformación en dióxido de carbono es más elevada en los microsomas hepáticos y renales de roedores (hámster, ratón, rata) que en los microsomas hepáticos y renales humanos. Además, el cloroformo se biotransforma más rápidamente en los microsomas renales del ratón que en los de la rata.

El hígado es el órgano vulnerable a la toxicidad aguda en las ratas y en varias estirpes de ratones. La lesión hepática se caracteriza principalmente por una infiltración grasa temprana y células con forma de globo y evoluciona hacia la necrosis centrilobular seguida de necrosis general. El riñón es el órgano vulnerable en los ratones macho de otras estirpes más sensibles. La lesión renal comienza con una degeneración hidrópica que avanza hacia la necrosis de los tubos proximales. No se ha observado una toxicidad renal apreciable en las ratas hembra de ninguna estirpe.

La toxicidad aguda varía según la raza, el sexo y el vehículo. En el ratón, la DL_{50} por vía oral oscila entre 36 y 1366 mg de cloroformo/kg de peso corporal, mientras que en las ratas oscila entre 450 y 2000 mg de cloroformo/kg de peso corporal. Después de una sola exposición de cuatro horas por inhalación, se observó toxicidad hepática en ratones y ratas cuando el nivel de cloroformo alcanzaba, respectivamente, 490 y 1410 mg/m^3.

Los efectos tóxicos del cloroformo más generales observados consisten en lesiones hepáticas. La gravedad de esos efectos por unidad de dosis administrada depende de la especie, del vehículo de administración y del método por el cual se haya administrado el cloroformo. La dosis más baja causante de lesión hepática observada es de 15 mg/kg de peso corporal por día, administrada a perros pachones en una base de pasta dentífrica durante un periodo de 7,5 años. No se han examinado efectos con dosis más bajas. Se necesitan dosis algo más elevadas para producir efectos hepatotóxicos en otras especies. En esos estudios, aunque la duración de la exposición variaba, los niveles sin efectos adversos observados oscilaban entre 15 y 125 mg/kg de peso corporal por día.

Se han observado efectos en el riñón de ratones macho de estirpes sensibles y en la rata F-344. Se han observado efectos graves en una estirpe especialmente sensible de ratones macho con dosis de sólo 36 mg/kg de peso corporal por día.

La inhalación de cloroformo seis horas por día durante siete días consecutivos produjo atrofia de las glándulas de Bowman y neoplasia ósea en la concha nasal de ratas F-344. El nivel en que no se observaron esos efectos fue de 14,7 mg/m^3 (3 ppm). La importancia de dichos efectos se está investigando más a fondo en estudios de larga duración.

El cloroformo administrado por sonda en un vehículo de aceite de maíz en dosis de 138 a 477 mg/kg de peso corporal por día indujo tumores hepáticos en ratones. Sin embargo, dosis semejantes de cloroformo administradas en el agua de bebida no produjeron tumores hepáticos en ratones. Por otra parte, en estudios de iniciación/promoción, el cloroformo administrado en el agua de bebida como promotor parecía inhibir el desarrollo de tumores hepáticos iniciados por dietilnitrosamina en ratones. Así pues, el vehículo y/o el método de administración del cloroformo es una variable importante en relación con la inducción de tumores hepáticos en el ratón.

El cloroformo administrado por sonda en aceite de maíz en dosis de 90 a 200 mg/kg de peso corporal por día indujo tumores renales en ratas. Sin embargo, en esa especie se observaron efectos semejantes tras la administración de cloroformo en el agua de bebida, lo que indica que la reacción no depende exclusivamente del vehículo utilizado.

Los efectos carcinogénicos del cloroformo en el hígado y los riñones de roedores parecen estar estrechamente relacionados con efectos citotóxicos y de replicación celular observados en los órganos vulnerables. Se ha observado que los efectos en la replicación celular eran paralelos a las modificaciones de las respuestas carcinogénicas al cloroformo inducidas por el vehículo y por la modalidad de administración. Las observaciones realizadas indican que el cloroformo tiene poca o ninguna capacidad para inducir mutaciones genéticas o daños directos de otro tipo en el ADN. Por otra parte, el cloroformo no parece poder iniciar tumores hepáticos en ratones ni de inducir síntesis imprevistas de ADN *in vivo*. Por otra parte, el cloroformo puede promover la neoplasia hepática cuando se administra en un vehículo oleoso. Por consiguiente, es probable que, tras la administración prolongada de cloroformo, la citotoxicidad seguida de proliferación celular sea la causa más importante del desarrollo de tumores hepáticos y renales en los roedores.

Algunos datos limitados sugieren que el cloroformo es tóxico para el feto, pero sólo en dosis tóxicas para la madre.

En general, el cloroformo provoca en el ser humano los mismos síntomas de toxicidad que en los animales. En el ser humano, la anestesia puede causar la muerte por arritmia e insuficiencia respiratoria y cardíaca. En el ser humano también se ha observado necrosis de los tubos renales y disfunción renal. Los niveles más bajos en los que se haya comunicado toxicidad hepática debida a la exposición ocupacional al cloroformo se sitúan entre 80 y 160 mg/m^3 (con un periodo de exposición inferior a cuatro meses) en un estudio y entre 10 y 1000 mg/m^3 (con periodos de exposición de uno a cuatro años) en otro estudio. La dosis letal media de un adulto se estima en unos 45 g, pero hay grandes diferencias de vulnerabilidad de un individuo a otro. En algunos estudios epidemiológicos hay ciertas indicaciones de que existe una asociación entre la exposición a los subproductos de la desinfección del agua de bebida y el cáncer colorrectal y de vejiga. Sin embargo, hay factores confusos y otras insuficiencias que ponen en entredicho esos estudios. Las pruebas de la carcinogenicidad del agua de bebida clorada en el ser humano son insuficientes. Además, los subproductos de la desinfección no pueden atribuirse al cloroformo por sí solo.

El cloroformo es tóxico en las fases embriolarvales de algunas especies de anfibios y de peces. La CL$_{50}$ más baja comunicada es de 0,3 mg/litro en las fases embriolarvales de *Hyla crucifer*. El cloroformo es menos tóxico para los peces y para *Daphnia magna*. La CL$_{50}$ de varias especies de peces se halla entre 18 y 191 mg/litro. Hay pocas diferencias de sensibilidad entre los peces de agua dulce y salada. La CL$_{50}$ más baja comunicada en *Daphnia magna* es de 29 mg/litro. El cloroformo es poco tóxico para las algas y otros microorganismos.

El Grupo Especial llegó a la conclusión de que los datos disponibles son suficientes para fijar una ingesta diaria tolerable sin efectos neoplásicos e ingestas con riesgos carcinogénicos específicos del cloroformo sobre la base de los estudios realizados en especies animales; las dosis servirán como orientación para que las autoridades competentes fijen límites de exposición. Sin embargo, se advierte que, cuando las circunstancias locales exijan optar entre el cumplimiento de límites microbiológicos y el de límites para subproductos de la desinfección tales como el cloroformo, debe siempre prevalecer la calidad microbiológica. *Nunca* debe comprometerse una desinfección eficaz.

Sobre la base del estudio de Heywood et al. (1979) en el cual se observó una ligera hepatotoxicidad (aumento de las enzimas del suero hepático y quistes grasos) en perros pachones que habían ingerido 15 mg/kg de peso corporal por día en pasta dentífrica durante 7,5 años, incorporando un factor de incertidumbre de 1000 (x10 para la variación entre especies, x10 para la variación dentro de la especie y x10 para utilizar un nivel con efectos en lugar de sin efectos y un estudio subcrónico), se obtiene una ingesta diaria tolerable (IDT) de 15 µg/kg de peso corporal por día.

En función de los datos disponibles sobre los mecanismos determinantes, el método que se considera más apropiado para establecer orientaciones fundadas en los tumores hepáticos de ratones es dividir un nivel sin efectos de proliferación celular por un factor de incertidumbre. A partir del nivel sin efectos observados de citoletalidad y proliferación celular en ratones B6C3F$_1$, de 10 mg/kg de peso corporal por día administrados en aceite de maíz durante tres semanas, comunicado en el estudio de Larson et al. (1993b), incorporando un factor de incertidumbre de 1000 (x10 para la variación entre especies, x10 para la variación dentro de la especie y x10 para la gravedad del efecto, es decir, carcinogenicidad, y estudio subcrónico) se obtiene una IDT de 10 µg/kg de peso corporal por día.

Se reconoce que los tumores renales en ratas también pueden estar asociados con letalidad y proliferación celular. Sin embargo, dado que no se dispone de datos sobre proliferación celular en la estirpe en la que se observaron tumores y la información sobre proliferación y letalidad celulares es de corto plazo (una sola sonda y exposición por inhalación durante siete días), se considera prematuro alejarse del modelo establecido por defecto (es decir, fases múltiples linearizadas) como base para estimar el riesgo de cáncer durante una vida. La ingesta diaria total que se considera asociada con un riesgo excesivo de 10^{-5} durante una vida, sobre la base de la inducción de tumores renales (adenomas y adenocarcinomas) en ratas macho en el estudio de Jorgenson et al. (1985), es de 8,2 µg/kg de peso corporal por día.

Los niveles de cloroformo en las aguas superficiales son generalmente bajos y no se prevé que constituyan un peligro para los organismos acuáticos. Sin embargo, niveles más elevados de cloroformo en las aguas superficiales como consecuencia de las descargas o los derrames industriales tal vez sean peligrosos en las fases embriolarvales de algunas especies acuáticas.

www.ingramcontent.com/pod-product-compliance
Lightning Source LLC
Chambersburg PA
CBHW031854200326
41597CB00012B/412